Terrorism, Trauma and Psychology

T0270704

This book provides a comprehensive insight into the multi-layered effects experienced by directly affected victims and their indirectly affected family members following terrorist incidents and other world disasters. Chapters draw primarily on interviews with 50 victims of the Bali bombings, but also consider terrorist incidents including the London and Boston bombings, and disasters such as the Boxing Day tsunami and the Fukushima nuclear disaster.

The book provides a detailed exploration of experiences and perceptions of those involved in the traumatic events, as well as their families, emergency response teams and community volunteers. Chapters discuss community responses to major incidents, appropriate non-medical models of intervention and vulnerable groups that may require special attention. The findings and analysis presented contribute to our understanding of the multi-layered effects of terrorism on victims of all levels, and the importance of a planned and informed response which includes the local community and its wealth of pre-existing resources.

Terrorism, Trauma and Psychology will be key reading for researchers and academics in the fields of social and clinical psychology, as well as scholars of victimology and terrorism studies.

Gwen Brookes is a psychologist in private practice, a member of the Australian Psychological Society, a research associate of Curtin University and an adjunct lecturer at the Department of Medicine and Pharmacology, Fremantle Unit at the University of Western Australia, Australia.

Julie Ann Pooley is the Associate Dean of Learning and Teaching in the Faculty of Health, Engineering and Science and an Associate Professor of Psychology in the School of Psychology and Social Science at Edith Cowan University, Australia.

Jaya Earnest is Director of Graduate Studies in the Faculty of Health Sciences and Associate Professor of International Health in the School of Nursing and Midwifery at Curtin University, Western Australia.

Explorations in Social Psychology series

Terrorism, Trauma and Psychology

A multilevel victim perspective of the Bali bombings

Gwen Brookes, Julie Ann Pooley and Jaya Earnest

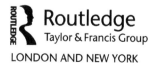

Routledge
Taylor & Francis Group

LONDON AND NEW YORK

First published 2015
by Routledge

2 Park Square, Milton Park, Abingdon, Oxfordshire OX14 4RN
711 Third Avenue, New York, NY 10017

Routledge is an imprint of the Taylor & Francis Group, an informa business

First issued in paperback 2017

British Library Cataloguing-in-Publication Data
A catalogue record for this book is available from the British
Library

Library of Congress Cataloging in Publication Data
Brookes, Gwen.
  Terrorism, trauma and psychology : a multilevel victim
  perspective of the Bali bombings / Gwen Brookes,
  Julie Ann Pooley and Jaya Earnest.
    pages cm. – (Explorations in social psychology series)
  1. Bali Bombings, Kuta, Bali, Indonesia, 2002. 2. Victims of
  terrorism–Psychology. 3. Psychic trauma. 4. Terrorism–
  Psychological aspects. I. Pooley, Julie Ann. II. Earnest, Jaya.
  III. Title.
  HV6433.I5B76 2015
  363.32509598'62–dc23   2014025866

ISBN: 978-1-138-78884-8 (hbk)
ISBN: 978-0-8153-5608-0 (pbk)

Typeset in Galliard
by Sunrise Setting Ltd, Paignton, UK

We dedicate this book to the 202 men and women from 21 countries who lost their lives in the 2002 Bali bombing, to the men and women interviewed for this study, to the many volunteer and professional responders who came together in a quest to help and to the thousands who continue to lose their lives in terrorist attacks globally.

Contents

Illustrations

Figures

Tables

Photographs

Preface

In the past decade terrorist attacks and suicide bombings have killed, injured and intimidated tens of thousands of people in many countries around the world. Trying to conceptualise the impact of terrorist events is difficult. However, attempting to understand, examine and discuss issues relevant to the individuals and communities who have experienced a terrorist attack helps contribute to a better understanding of why these events occur in the first place. More importantly, it also helps to process the impact of the events for individuals and communities that are in the course of moving forward. This book is the result of an exploratory, qualitative study undertaken in the aftermath of the Bali bombings that took place in 2002, when two bombs were deliberately exploded by terrorists in the Sari nightclub and Paddy's bar in the popular tourist area of Kuta, Bali, Indonesia.

In the period of time that followed the initial attack it is fair to say that the direct victims, their family members and their communities were traumatised, confused and frightened. The period that this book charts runs from the initial aftermath of the attack to six years later, when most of the physical wounds had healed but the legacy of the attacks remained very real to those who were witness to them. This book describes the experiences, and tries to understand the perspectives, of two particular groups of people: the Balinese community and, from the Australian perspective, the Perth community who were visiting Bali at the time of the attack in Kuta.

The study was conducted in Bali and Perth in 2008. The overarching aim was to examine the multi-layered effects and forms of support received by victims and their family members in the aftermath of the 2002 bombings and in the period after. Further to this, exploration of the perceptions and experiences of the Indonesian and Australian emergency response teams and community volunteers who assisted in the aftermath of the crisis was important. In addition, a systematic review was carried out of the available literature examining the multi-layered effects of terrorist attacks and natural disasters – including the London (2005) and Boston (2013) bombings, the Boxing Day tsunami (2005) and the Fukushima nuclear disaster (2011) – and the forms of post-attack disaster support offered to victims and their families. In bringing together understandings from the literature, the experiences of victims, members of response teams and community volunteers, it becomes possible to propose a list of recommendations that may be useful to professionals and non-professionals in the aftermath of these events.

The conceptual framework for the study was based on the work of the Psychosocial Working Group (PWG) (2003), who developed a framework to identify the complex needs of individuals and communities in the aftermath of disasters in order to promote strategies for good practice for external support agencies. The framework contains three dimensions which help people cope in the aftermath of a disaster. The first dimension is **human capacity** (encompassing the skills and knowledge of the people); the second is **social ecology** (encompassing familial, religious and cultural resources); and the final dimension is **culture and values** (encompassing cultural values, beliefs and practices).

The framework was modified in this study to help with examination of the participant responses. The modified framework was used to help identify specific key themes and resources used for support during the bombings and those that had been depleted as a result of the bombings. Data specific to the multi-layered effects of the bombing was defined as 'disrupted resources' and data which referred to the types of support participants received in the aftermath as 'reinforced resources'. A full exploration of the framework and its use in the current study is in chapter 3 of this book.

For this study 50 participants were identified, using snowball and purposive recruiting strategies, including 33 participants from the Balinese community in Indonesia and 17 participants from the Perth community in Western Australia. This qualitative case-study approach allowed each participant to share their stories and reflect on the multi-layered effects they experienced. Importantly, this qualitative study incorporates the voices of the 50 participants, which are woven throughout the chapters.

Overall, in both Bali and Perth, victims at all levels reported many symptoms of distress in the initial aftermath of the bombings. Most of the effects reported could be termed normal distress reactions to a very abnormal event. The poor economic situation in Bali appeared to compound the effects for many of the Balinese victims: as a result of the attack, many of the injured and their families were left almost destitute. A number of victims described reactions such as depression, suicidal ideation and fear during thunderstorms and the many cultural celebrations on the island. There were many similarities in effects uncovered across victim groups in both countries, especially in terms of the intense emotions described following the loss of a loved one or injury.

In Bali and Perth, primary-level victims described the importance of practical, economic, emotional and spiritual support from their families and the community. The tales of 'mateship' and families and communities responding to help were many, and offered an invaluable and unique insight into this disaster. In addition, the study highlighted the crucial role played by the many volunteer and professional responders in the initial aftermath of an attack. The study highlighted how many victims also experience adverse reactions such as emotional numbing and derealisation. For most it was a temporary and understandable reaction to the difficult tasks they had to undertake.

Although the focus of the study was a terrorist attack, the recommendations can be considered in reference to other forms of complex emergencies. They have been listed in a framework – to be found in chapter 8 of this book – that is intended for use by professionals, non-professionals and agencies involved in responding in the aftermath of complex emergencies. The aim of these recommendations is to enable professionals, non-professionals, governments and agencies to be more informed and prepared.

The Bali disaster revealed the strength of the human spirit, resilience and the willingness of people and countries to help each other in times of extreme distress and need. It also highlighted aspects of response which could be improved. This information and study is offered in a collegial manner to add to the existing experience and knowledge in the complex emergency arena. It is intended to encourage a psychosocial response to any disaster situation, based on the knowledge that communities have pre-existing resources which can and should be utilised in these difficult circumstances.

Acknowledgements

We would like to thank the following people for helping with this project:

First and foremost, we thank the participants interviewed in Bali and Perth for their generosity in sharing their journeys.

Thank you to the staff and management of YKIDS and YKIP in Bali and to the board of Kingsley Football Club, in particular Amanda McIlroy and Jan Pearce, who gave their support to the study.

To Sherlyana Putru and Ketut Cakra, two very special research assistants in Bali, for their patience, diligence and cultural knowledge.

To Dr Alison Strang, senior research fellow at the Institute for International Health and Development, Queen Margaret University and Professor Alistair Ager at the Mailman School of Public Health, Columbia University Medical Center, for their support and sharing of their psychosocial methodological framework.

On a personal note, none of this could be done without thank-yous to Gwen's family, Denis, Caroline, Jonathan and Valerie, and also to Florence (1) and Archie (4), her lovely grandchildren, and her friends Marg, Caroline, Hilary, Marie, Tina, and Julie; to Julie Ann's family, Peter, Charlotte and Samantha; and to Jaya's family, especially her mum Maria.

Gwen Brookes, Julie Ann Pooley and Jaya Earnest

Abbreviations

ABC	Australian Broadcasting Corporation
ABS	Australian Bureau of Statistics
ADB	Asian Development Bank
AFL	Australian Rules Football League
AFP	Australian Federal Police
AGD	Australian Government Directory
ARC	Australian Research Council
ARI	Asia Research Institute
ARISE	A Relational Sequence of Engagement
BBC	British Broadcasting Corporation
BIWA	Bali International Women's Association
CISD	Centre for the Study of Traumatic Stress
CNN	Cable News Network
DCD	Department of Community Development
DFAT	Australian Department of Foreign Affairs and Trade
EFRJ	European Forum for Restorative Justice
GDP	Gross Domestic Product
HEARTS	History, Emotions, Asking, Reason and Teaching Model
IASC	Inter-agency Standing Committee
ICU	Intensive Care Unit
IMF	International Monetary Fund
IR	Indonesian Rupiah
IRA	Irish Republican Army
IRC	International Red Cross
JI	Jemaah Islamiyah
KAFC	Kingsley Amateur Football Club
KI	Key Informant
LTTE	Liberation Tigers of Tamil Eelam
NGO	Non-government Organisation
NSECRH	National Statement on Ethical Conduct in Research involving Humans
PFA	Psychological First Aid
PIJ	Palestine Islamic Jihad

PLO	Palestine Liberation Organisation
PLV	Primary-level Victims
PM	Prime Minister
PTG	Post-traumatic Growth
PTSD	Post-traumatic Stress Disorder
PWB	Psychosocial Well-being
PWG	Psychosocial Working Group
SLV	Secondary-level Victim
SMI	Severe Mental Illness
SSNP	Syrian Social Nationalist Party
TFR	Total Fertility Rate
THK	*Tri Hita Karana*
USAID	United States Agency for International Development
UDF	Ulster Defence Force
UN	United Nations
UNAMI	United Nations Assistance Mission for Iraq
UNDP	United Nations Development Programme
UNOCHA	United Nations Office for the Co-ordination of Humanitarian Affairs
UVF	Ulster Volunteer Force
WAFL	West Australian Rules Football League
WHO	World Health Organization
WMD	Weapons of Mass Destruction
WTF	War Trauma Foundation
WVI	World Vision International
YKIDS	Yayasan Kuta International Disaster Scholarship
YKIP	Yayasan Kemanusiaan Ibu Pertiwi

Chapter 1

Introduction

Overview of the chapter

The primary focus of this chapter is to present an overview of the history of terrorism, as it is an important adjunct to our understanding of the concept, motives and rationale of terrorism. Further to this, the political and other objectives of terrorist attacks are discussed, as is the nature of terrorism – especially in countries which have experienced protracted conflict, such as Israel/Palestine, Afghanistan, Somalia, the Democratic Republic of Congo (DRC) and Sri Lanka. The chapter concludes with a discussion surrounding the possible future of terrorism and terrorist organisations, and then finally introduces the context of the study – the island of Bali.

Background to the study

Modern terrorism

Events such as 9/11, the Bali bombing, the Mumbai attacks and the recent Boston bombings can easily lead to the view that terrorism is a modern-day phenomenon; yet when we look back historically, we see terrorism has been in existence for a long period of time. Terrorist acts have been designed to frighten and intimidate the many by targeting the few, and terrorism has probably existed for millennia (Miller, 2004). It is even said to have existed as far back as 66–73 AD, with reports of assassinations occurring throughout Roman history. During this period, many brutal acts were carried out in crowded places, designed to create the same type of fear and reactions that modern-day terrorists attempt to produce, such as elements of political unrest (Gearson, 2002). By examining terrorism through the ages we add to our understanding of the concept, motives and rationale behind terrorist acts.

There is little difference between historical and modern-day terrorism: all suicide attacks or assassination attempts come with a degree of what is termed 'psychological toxicity' (Dougall *et al*, 2005, p. 28), as the 'many are intimidated by the actions of a few'. Relatively recent events such as the Bali attacks in 2002 and

2005, the Madrid train bombings in March 2004[1] and the Mumbai attacks in November 2008[2] share a commonality in that they targeted, killed and injured many people, and instilled fear in the rest of the population. The attacks involved few operatives and were random and unexpected in nature, with the perpetrators all claiming to be members of radical Islamic groups. Despite what the popular press would have its readers believe, Islamic terrorism is only one of many forms of terrorism: other forms include suicide terrorism, economic terrorism, domestic terrorism, international terrorism and bio-terrorism. As modern terrorism appears to have many aims and facets, it is difficult to define, and many definitions can be found.

On close examination, three main characteristics emerge which are common to all definitions: the intention to cause death or serious injury, particularly to non-combatant civilians; the intention to cause damage to infrastructure and property; and a desire to intimidate a government or population (Michael and Scolnick, 2006; Sheppard, 2009). Consideration of the Madrid train bombings, the London underground and bus bombings[3] and the Mumbai attacks reveals all of these aims were achieved, and to great effect.

Global terrorist attacks

In recent years, terrorist attacks have occurred in numerous countries across the globe. Between 1994 and 2003 there were 32 terrorist attacks in 39 countries, resulting in 3,299 deaths (Wilson and Thomson, 2005). The Global Terrorism Index (GTI) from 2002 to 2011 highlights that global terrorism significantly and steadily increased, particularly in the 2005 to 2007 period. This increase is demonstrated by examining the terrorist incidents which occurred in just one year, 2011, in which 4,564 global incidents resulted in 7,473 deaths and 13,961 injuries. These attacks are usually extremely well planned and, for the first time in recent history, non-combatant civilians are the primary target of violence (Winkates, 2006) – as opposed to the two World Wars, when professional soldiers and strategic buildings were usually the targets. This is highlighted by the number of attacks on military institutions in the period 2002–2011, which accounted for only 4 per cent of terrorist incidents (Institute for Economics and Peace, 2012).

The classic example of a modern-day terrorist event is the attacks of 11 September 2001 (9/11) in New York, Washington and Pennsylvania. In these attacks, 19 terrorists hijacked four airliners and crashed them into the twin towers of the World Trade Center in New York, the Pentagon in Washington and a field in Pennsylvania. The 9/11 attacks were the largest human-made disaster on American soil, with approximately 3,000 individuals reported killed and many thousands more injured (DeLisi et al, 2003). The terrorists had deliberately set out to kill themselves and as many other non-combatant civilians as possible. The fear this act instilled in the American public, and the world, was immeasurable.

In the following year, 2002, the Indonesian island of Bali was targeted. At 11.08 pm on Saturday 12 October in Legian Street, Kuta, a popular bar, Paddy's, was targeted by a suicide bomber. Tourists and locals ran outside to escape the heat and turmoil that resulted in the explosion. At 11.17 pm a larger bomb secreted in a panel van outside the Sari club was detonated. The bombings resulted in a large fire, which engulfed approximately 200 metres of Legian Street. Many tourists and locals in the vicinity of Legian Street and inside the bar and club were killed and injured. The casualties amounted to 202 deceased and 325 injured (Yayasan IDEP, 2003).

In October 2005, Bali was again targeted by suicide bombers when terrorists exploded two bombs in Kuta and one in Jimbaran Bay, resulting in 23 fatalities ('Australia's emergency response', 2005). On both occasions, Australian tourists were among the fatalities. The attacks were perpetrated by suicide bombers who perfected the technique of quietly infiltrating deep into their enemies' territory without drawing attention to themselves, which is a technique that allows for low security risks (Ramasubramanian, 2004) for the terrorist embedded in the targeted community. The effect of these attacks on primary-level victims was extensive, both physically and psychologically.

The 9/11 attacks of 2001 and the London bombings in 2005 were also perpetrated by suicide attackers. Although such events are relatively small in number, suicide bombings have contributed to the fear and terror individuals and communities feel following terrorist attacks. Suicide attacks account for 48 per cent of the terror attack death statistics worldwide and have been termed the most aggressive form of terrorism (Pape, 2003). They are a difficult concept to understand as, according to Pastor (2004, p. 701), suicide terrorism 'defies a basic psychological drive – the need for self-preservation'. Yet many terrorists are ready to sacrifice their own lives 'in the process of destroying or attempting to destroy a target to advance a political goal' (Jane's Intelligence review, cited in Winkates, 2006, p. 89), and as one terrorist dies another, it seems, is ready and willing to take their place.

The objectives of terrorism

Apart from killing mainly non-combatant civilians and causing general fear and unrest in the community, one of the primary aims of terrorism is to achieve an intense political objective (Ramsubramanian, 2004; Winkates, 2006). For example, on 11 March 2004 a series of ten terrorist bombs were detonated on early-morning rush-hour trains in Madrid, Spain. A total of 191 commuters were killed and 1,800 injured, and the incident was declared Europe's worst-ever terrorist attack (*USA Today*, 2007). The objective in this instance appeared to be political, as the bombings occurred just three days before the Spanish general election. At the election, the previously popular ruling conservative-leaning party was voted out of office. Connections appeared to have been made by the Spanish voters to the Aznar government's open support for the war in Iraq and the deployment of Spanish troops in Afghanistan (Powell, 2004). The Spanish Socialist Workers' Party was brought to power with a pledge to withdraw all troops from Afghanistan, which they did shortly after winning office. It seemed the bombers had achieved their objective.

Terrorist attacks are not new to Spain, as the Basque separatist movement has been operating in the country since 1959 with the aim of forcing the government to allow separation of the greater Basque region. In 2009 it was suspected of planting a bomb which killed two Spanish policemen on the holiday island of Mallorca (Mielniezuk, 2009). Other countries have also endured long-standing disputes and terrorist attacks, and these will now be discussed.

Nations which have experienced protracted conflict and terrorist attacks

Sri Lanka

The popular press portrays suicide bombers as mainly belonging to fundamental Islamic groups, yet it is the predominantly Hindu Tamil group that has been listed as the world leader in suicide terrorism (Ramasubramanian, 2004). The civil war in Sri Lanka lasted from 1983 to 2009 and resulted in the loss of 60,000 lives and 800,000 displaced persons (Goodhand *et al*, 2011). Over a 30-year period the Liberation Tigers of Tamil Eelam (LTTE), commonly known as the Tamil Tigers, agitated for a homeland for ethnic Tamils. The Tamils waged a war against the Sinhalese majority who make up 90 per cent of the population in Sri Lanka and are thought to have pioneered the use of the suicide jacket, as well as the use of women in lone suicide attacks (Bhattacharji, 2008). Whether using male or female suicide bombers, suicide attacks were a fundamental part of the LTTE's strategy in their fight for separatism. They are the only group to have effectively used suicide missions to assassinate two world leaders, namely Rajiv Gandhi of India in 1991 and President Ranasinghe Premadasa of Sri Lanka in 1993 (Ramasubramanian, 2004).

Sri Lanka is one of a small number of countries in which suicide terrorism became a regular occurrence and a major strategic threat (Moghadam, 2003). There was never a shortage of volunteers willing to become suicide bombers: 273 men and women were reported to have taken up the role up to 2006. To mark the esteem suicide bombers attracted in their community in Kilinochchi, a Tamil stronghold, the 'martyrdom' of their many suicide bombers was marked by 5 July being named 'black tiger day' in their honour (Mitchell, 2006).

The Israeli–Palestinian conflict

The West Bank cities, the Gaza strip and Israel's borders and land divisions have been a focus for occupation and conflict between the Israeli and Palestinian people for many years. The more recent Palestinian and Israeli conflicts began in December 1987 and have continued in cycles up to the present day. The Israelis have con-trolled the West Bank for 22 years, having made a withdrawal from the Gaza strip in 2005. According to a United Nations special paper, between the beginning of a new cycle of conflict in 2000 and July 2007, at least 5,845 people died in the conflict, of whom 4,250 were Palestinian and 1,024 Israeli. For every person killed, approximately seven were injured. Most of those killed had not been involved in the fighting and were therefore civilians; 1,497 of the dead were children, and 626 were women (United Nations Office for the Coordination of Humanitarian Affairs [UNOCHA], 2007). Unfortunately, this conflict has resulted in death and injury to many non-combatant citizens of both countries, who are caught up in the dangerous political war that unfolds as they go about their daily business.

An aspect of that war is the use of suicide bombings, which occur frequently in Israel. The suicide bombers are almost always highly mobile and organised. They have carried out attacks on civilian targets in places such as shopping malls, cafés, buses and holiday resorts. These missions have been undertaken in most of the major towns and cities of Israel (Kaplan *et al*, 2006), and challenge citizens' notions of personal safety and freedom from fear. This is a challenge the citizens of Israel have endured for many years: between 2001 and 2014, 1,241 civilians were killed and 8,549 injured as a direct result of terrorism (Israel Ministry of Foreign Affairs, 2014). Although there are fewer suicide bombings now, in the past they have been the leading cause of death in Israel (Kaplan *et al*, 2006). This particular method is still used as a fear tactic by Palestinian groups in an attempt to persuade Israel to move out of the West Bank. It is a popular method of attack, as the body suits worn by the suicide bombers are difficult to detect but cheap and easy to make and conceal.

The conflict in Iraq

The United States invaded Iraq in 2003, with the intention of assisting Iraq in becoming a democracy and as part of the American-inspired 'Global War on Terrorism'. Iraq has instead become a country pervaded by a civil war between Sunni and Shiite Muslims and by terrorist attacks (Galbraith, 2006). According to a United Nations Assistance Mission Report (United Nations, 2006), it is estimated that in 2006 civilian deaths numbered 34,452 and the number of civilians injured amounted to 36,685. Suicide missions have become almost a daily occurrence in Iraq, where they have been utilised as a strategic weapon to persuade US and other foreign troops to return home or to interfere with people's right to vote in a general election.

One example from the many such tragic events in Iraq is that of a suicide bomber who killed at least 28 people by detonating a suicide belt outside a police recruitment centre in Baghdad (BBC News, 2009). The terrorists usually aim to detonate their bombs in crowded areas, to increase the number of civilian casualties and to cause the maximum amount of community fear and unrest. As most terrorist attacks are designed to kill and injure innocent people and instil fear in the populace, suicide bombings of any type appear to be a quick and economic method of achieving a deadly objective.

Despite a number of suicide bombings and continued threats of violence, Iraq held democratic elections in March 2010. Ayad Allawi's Iraqiya party won a majority share of the vote, yet no single party achieved an outright majority. Mr Allawai indicated that all attempts to build a united government have failed, and that this may lead to more political unrest, violence and even a new sectarian war (Chulov, 2010). Certainly, the suicide bombings did not abate: for example, at least five were killed and 40 wounded in a roadside car bombing near a provincial council member's house in Northern Iraq on 19 June 2010 (Mahmoud, 2010). Elections were held again in April 2013, with more than 21 million registered voters and more than 9,000 candidates vying for their support. Again it was expected that no one party would be elected when the final results were announced on 25 May (*The Economist*, 2014). The unrest and violence has continued, with an estimated 7,800 people, mostly civilians, killed in 2013. The continuing unrest between the majority Shi'a and minority Sunni population continues to fuel violence across the country (*The Economist*, 2014).

It is difficult to predict the future for Iraq. US President Barack Obama confirmed an election campaign promise in 2009 to initiate a staged withdrawal of American troops: it was proposed that the number of troops would be reduced to almost one third by August 2010, with a total withdrawal planned by the end of December 2010 (De Young, 2009). In fact it was on 18 December 2011 that the final squadron of troops left Iraq. At the most violent stage of the war, some 170,000 US troops were stationed in 500 bases in Iraq. Almost 4,500 US soldiers were killed and many more wounded. In addition, tens of thousands of Iraqis have died since the US-led campaign began in 2003. Apart from the huge loss of life, it has also been a costly commitment for America: by the war's end it had cost the US almost A$1 trillion (BBC News, 2011).

In a serious turn of events commencing on 10 June 2014 the unrest in Iraq escalated, with the Islamic State of Iraq and the Levant (ISIL) militants advancing across the country in an attempt to overthrow the government with the overall aim of establishing a Sunni state (Cooper, 2014), which may end in a full-scale civil war. It is reported they are marching south towards Baghdad and, as always, civilians are being caught up in the conflict, with many thousands reportedly trying to flee to safer regions such as autonomous Kurdistan (Cooper, 2014). A recent UN media report (August 2014) confirms ISIL has made many inroads into Northern Iraq, with many thousands of civilians, particularly the ethnic and vulnerable minorities of Christians, Turkomen and Yezidis continuing to be displaced. This has produced a dangerous humanitarian crisis, with many thousands of Yezidis amassing along the Turkish border and in the Sinjar mountains, with little shelter, food or water. International communities have responded by dropping urgently required supplies by air.

In addition to this displacement, many thousands of others who are in minority groups or oppose the ideology of ISIL are being ruthlessly killed by armed militants (UN Media Report, 2014). The American response has been guarded thus far, with President Obama ordering limited airstrikes on ISIL positions near the Kurdish capital of Erbil in an effort to protect the large contingent of American personnel positioned there as advisors and embassy staff. He has also ordered humanitarian aid drops in the Sinjar mountain region to help alleviate the large humanitarian crisis which is evolving (Cooper *et al*, 2014). Quite how the international community will interpret and respond to UN Secretary-General Mr Ban Ki-moon's call for the international community, 'especially those with influence and resources, to positively impact the situation' (UN Media Report, 2014, p. 1) will be interesting to see.

The protracted conflict in Afghanistan

Afghanistan has been in a state of protracted conflict in the past decades, with civil war, the war with the former USSR, Taliban rule and the War on Terror. The first of these conflicts started in 1978 when the Saur Revolution overthrew the government and killed civilians. This was followed by opposition of the Mujahedeen, a battle which lasted for the next 11 years and resulted in two million deaths and 1.5 million injured civilians. Almost half of the population were displaced: 1.5 million Afghans moved to Pakistan and Iran respectively as refugees, and countryside residents were forced to live in Kabul (UN News Centre, 2014).

The Taliban, an armed Islamic conservative group shaped in 1990, took control of Kabul with the vast financial support of Osama bin Laden and ruled the country in accordance with a very strict version of Islam. Examples of their changes to the norms and culture included forcing women to cover their face and full body, decreeing that women did not have the right to go out of the house without a related male or access education and banning music and dance. The Taliban government collapsed in 2001 due to US-led attacks on its bases in an attempt to find Osama bin Laden, whose Al Qaeda terrorist group claimed responsibility for the 9/11 attacks.

In 2013, the United Nations Assistance Mission in Afghanistan (UNAMA) documented that there had been 8,615 civilian casualties (2,959 civilian deaths and 5,656 injured) that year, marking increases of 7 per cent in deaths, 17 per cent in injured and 14 per cent in total civilian casualties compared to 2012. Suicide and bomb attacks resulted in 1,236 civilian casualties (255 killed and 981 injured) from 73 incidents in 2013. Conflict-related violence caused 746 women casualties (235 women killed and 511 injured), up 36 per cent from 2012, and child casualties increased by 34 per cent compared to 2012, to 1,756, with 561 children killed and 1,195 injured (United Nations Assistance Mission in Afghanistan, 2014).

Taliban attacks increased after 2006 and the UN estimates that they are the most common cause of civilian casualties in Afghanistan. The US planned to withdraw its army from Afghanistan and shift control to Afghan forces, but difficulties in training forces and high prevalence of drug use among troops has made this a difficult transition (Peace Direct, 2013). In 2013 the Taliban claimed responsibility for 153 attacks affecting civilians, an increase of 292 per cent compared to 2012. Most of these attacks either used indiscriminate tactics, such as IED detonations in public areas, or directly targeted civilians – particularly civilian administration personnel and buildings (United Nations Assistance Mission in Afghanistan, 2014).

On 27 May 2014, President Obama announced what appeared to be a final plan for a staged withdrawal of troops, with the aim that by the end of 2014 'America's combat role will be over in Afghanistan' (Obama, 2014, p. 1) and the Afghan police and military will be responsible for the security of their country. The number of troops in the country is to be reduced from 32,000 in 2014 to 9,800 by the beginning of 2015, with their activities primarily consisting of sharing a NATO peacekeeping role. By the end of 2016, it is planned that the normal squad of military personnel required to guard the American embassy in Kabul will be present (Obama, 2014). Even though the UN doubled its services to the Afghan people in the 1990s, rates of maternal and infant mortality continue to be among the highest in the world. UNHCR's attempts to return 4.6 million Afghan refugees to their homes remains a difficult task, especially given the presence of 9.7 million landmines in the ground (UN News Centre, 2014).

Somalia – a failed state

Following the downfall of President Siad Barre in 1991, civil war broke out in Somalia between the faction supporting Interim President Ali Mahdi Mohamed and that supporting General Mohamed Farah Aidid. The war resulted in nearly one million refugees and almost five million people threatened by hunger and disease. Since 1991, an estimated 350,000–1,000,000 Somalis have died as a result of the conflict, and up to 3,000 African Union soldiers have been killed fighting the Islamist insurgency in Somalia over the past few years (Chevigney, 2007).

Drawing on an extended Somalia Civil War report (n.d.), several distinctive phases of the conflict in the country can be defined:

- The period **1991–1992** was marked by intense conflict, as different clan factions fought for control of land and resources. This resulted in the devastation of inter-riverine areas, causing famine and disruption to farming and livestock production. Increasing numbers of refugees left the country for Kenya and Ethiopia. In 1991, the formation of independent Somaliland in the northwest created an enclave of relative peace (Somalia Civil War, n.d.).
- The period **1992–1995** centred on UN and US interventions. This phase was affected by localised conflicts, specifically around Mogadishu. Fighting among rival factions resulted in the killing, dislocation and starvation of thousands of Somalis, and led the United Nations to intervene militarily: in 1992, responding to the political chaos and humanitarian disaster in the

country, the United States and other nations launched peacekeeping operations. On 3 October 1993, the US suffered a significant number of casualties (19 Marines dead and over 80 others wounded) in a battle with Somali gunmen. The United States and UN withdrew their forces from Somalia in 1994 and 1995 (Somalia Civil War, n.d.).

- The period **1995–2000** was a post-intervention phase that witnessed the continued dissolution of the Somali state. Conflict between rival warlords and their factions continued throughout the 1990s. No stable government emerged to take control of the country. The UN assisted Somalia with food aid, but did not send peacekeeping troops into the country. Puntland, in the northeast, declared itself a regional administration in 1998 (Somalia Civil War, n.d.).

- The period **2000–2006** began with the establishment of the Transitional National Government (TNG) in Djibouti. Key warlords in Somalia continue to oppose the TNG, leading to conflict and further population displacement. In January 2004 the warlords reached a power-sharing agreement after talks in Kenya. The TNG was succeeded by the Transitional Federal Government (TFG), the 14th attempt at a government since 1991. The Islamic courts also emerged during this phase (Somalia Civil War, n.d.).

- The period **2006–2011** was marked by the December 2006 intervention of Ethiopian troops, which by January 2007 had dispersed the Islamic courts. However, the militant terrorist group **Al-Shabaab** emerged during this period and continued to fight against the TFG and foreign forces, and by 2008 it had gained control of Southern Somalia. In October 2011, at the invitation of the Somali Transitional Federal Government, the Kenyan government launched operations against Al-Shabaab, though the TNG was installed in Mogadishu (Somalia Civil War, n.d.).

After the attacks of 11 September 2001, the United States gradually began to take a more active role in Somalia's affairs, fearing that the country had become a haven for terrorists. The United States has strengthened engagement with the governments of Puntland and Somaliland as part of a two-track policy aimed at curbing the growth of terrorist extremism (Somalia Civil War, n.d.).

The world's deadliest conflict: the Democratic Republic of Congo (former Zaire)

Described as the world's deadliest conflict, the conflict in the DRC (formerly known as Zaire) has involved seven nations. Since the outbreak of fighting in August 1998, some 5.4 million people have died and 1.5 million continue to be displaced. The vast majority have actually died from malaria, diarrhoea, pneumonia and malnutrition – conditions which are typically preventable in normal circumstances, but were exacerbated because of the conflict. Children account for 47 per cent of the deaths (Shah, 2010).

The cruel irony in the DRC is that influential world nations benefit from the vast mineral resources of the country, especially diamonds. The main fighting has been on the eastern side of the DRC, with approximately 90 per cent of the DRC's internally displaced population having fled violence from that region. It is estimated there are more than one million internally displaced persons in the country's four eastern regions (Shah, 2010). It is reported that

> in October 2008, the situation in the east of the country worsened significantly as fighting and displacement sharply increased in the North Kivu province following an advance by rebel fighters led by Laurent Nkunda; according to the International Crisis Group (ICG, 2013), the army was implicated in looting, rapes and killings in and around the capital Goma as government troops abandoned their positions. In early November 2008, the UN accused the rebel forces and pro-government militias of having committed war crimes. In an attempt to bring the situation under control, in January 2009 the DRC government invited troops from Rwanda to help mount a joint operation against the Rwandan rebel Hutu militias active in eastern DR Congo
> (RULAC Project, 2014)

Hirsch and Wolfe (2012) state that mineral resources (especially diamonds) were being plundered with impunity and that there had been a new surge of rapes and killings. They say UN forces supporting Congolese government troops had failed to stop supply lines to Rwandan Hutu rebels. In 2012, 578 children, including 26 girls, were recruited into armed rebel forces and, as a direct result of conflict-related violence, 154 children (including 86 boys and 64 girls) were killed and 113 (including 76 boys and 35 girls) injured. During the reporting period 185 girls, most of whom were between 15 and 17 years of age, were subjected to rape or other forms of sexual violence. In the same year, 1,497 children (1,334 boys and 163 girls) were separated or escaped from armed rebel groups (UN Secretary-General Report, 2013).

While these protracted conflicts may seem somewhat unrelated to the issue of terrorist attacks per se, they provide opportunities for terrorist organisations to capitalise on the instability in countries and regions. The spill-over effects of civil and protracted conflicts impact local communities and sometimes also other countries, in which citizens reside as they have left their country of origin, possibly because of the conflict.

Modern terrorism and terrorist organisations

In his seminal assessment of terrorist organisations and methods post-9/11, Hoffman (2003) predicted: 'the image captured today is not the same as yesterday nor will it be the same as tomorrow' (p. 439). In other words, terrorist organisations and methods will continue to evolve and change. An example of this change can be seen in the terrorist attacks in Mumbai in 2008, in which a well co-ordinated, trained group of young men from Pakistan almost simultaneously attacked 12 strategic targets across the city, including two luxury hotels and the headquarters of a Jewish outreach group (Shekhar, 2009). On this occasion the terrorists were not suicide bombers, but men who were heavily armed with machine guns and grenades and who used military tactics to strike at the targets. The aim was to kill as many victims as possible and the terrorists were prepared to die for their cause.

The 2009 terrorist attacks in Jakarta saw tactics change again, possibly in an attempt to overcome already tight security. In this attack suicide bombers returned to the scene of a previous attack in 2003. They posed as legitimate guests and embedded themselves in the general day-to-day life of hotel guests of the JW Marriott and Ritz Carlton hotels. The terrorists appear to have manufactured their bombs in the hotels and detonated them in the hotel restaurants early one morning as people were eating breakfast (Jerard *et al*, 2009). It is clear is that in order to respond to the modern terrorist, the military and other organisations must be prepared and think outside the box, as terrorists continue to adopt non-conventional methods of attack. As Mishal and Rosenthal (2005, p. 290) state, they need to 'focus on an organisation that uses non-conventional tactics [and] may be fragmentised, de-territorialised, have fast moving operational capability and [use the] infinitive associative connections of Al Qaeda'.

In another attack by Taliban terrorists on 10 June 2014, ten gunmen broke through security at the international airport in Karachi, Pakistan and entered into an all-night siege which resulted in 34 deaths. In a surprise additional attack two days later, Taliban gunmen on motorbikes attacked an airport security training establishment. No one was injured in this attack and the gunmen fled after counterattacks by airport security staff and the military. The overall intent appeared to be political and aimed at disrupting the important peace talks between the Pakistani Prime Minister, his government and the Taliban. It also disrupted many flights and caused chaos in a very busy airport. In retaliation, the Pakistani air force attacked Taliban positions on the border with Afghanistan and killed 25 militants (Hassan, 2014). These particular attacks would seem to support the notion that the Pakistani Taliban share a similar ideology with the Afghan Taliban, but their primary focus is toppling the state of Pakistan and enforcing Islamic laws in the country (Hassan, 2014).

State-sponsored terrorism

In contemporary society, the word 'terrorist' is usually used for religiously motivated groups such as Al Qaeda, Hamas and Hezbollah. Between May 2003 and May 2004 terrorist acts were recorded in 54 countries of the world and on every continent bar Antarctica (US State Department, 2003), with many of these attacks being attributed to the groups mentioned above. A review of the literature, however, suggests that it is not only terrorist organisations that perpetrate terrorist acts. Rolston and Gilmartin (2000, p. 10) highlight how in their view the British government sanctioned the killings or, as they state it, 'assassinations of insurgents'.

These authors accuse the British government of involvement in, among others, the killing of a Northern Ireland solicitor who defended members of the IRA in court, drive-by shootings in Republican areas and many other acts of what could be termed 'state terrorism'. They believe acts of terrorism can be perpetrated by 'any kind or person, or organisation or state' and additionally highlight the use of state-sponsored terror squads in Uganda who were reported to have murdered 'tens of thousands of people' (2000, p. 12). The terror squads were part of Idi Amin's regime (1971–1979), which targeted the Acholi and Langi people, and in particular those in the armed forces (Tripp, 2004).

The recurring conflicts in Gaza have resulted in worldwide condemnation of the Israeli policy of collective punishment of Palestinians living in Gaza in retaliation for the Hamas rocket attacks on towns in Israel. At present there are no clear accusations of state terrorism; however, the statistics as highlighted may speak for themselves. In 2009 the International Red Cross (IRC) and UNOCHA reported 1,314 Palestinians had been killed in the conflict (412 of them children), with more than 5,300 injured, 21,000 houses destroyed and 50,000 people displaced (Holmes, 2009). During the Israeli bombing hospitals were also targeted, with 13 medical staff killed alongside seven UN staff. The continuing blockade of Gaza by the Israeli government also causes extreme difficulties for the citizens of Gaza. The humanitarian crisis caused by the bombings and blockade is difficult to imagine, as is the grief, loss and trauma experienced by all concerned. A 2008 Oxfam report captured the essence of the crisis:

> This humanitarian crisis is a direct result of on-going collective punishment of ordinary men, women and children and is illegal under international law. Isolation and poverty are breeding increasing levels of violence for which Palestinians and Israelis are paying the price.
>
> (Oxfam, 2008, p. 6)

Israel's ongoing punishment of the people of Gaza continues: a flotilla of ships carrying 10,000 tonnes of humanitarian aid designed to ease the blockade to Gaza was attacked in international waters by Israeli forces in March 2010 and a number of passengers were taken to Israel and forcibly detained prior to deportation. There were reports of armed Israeli troops boarding a number of the ships, resulting in 19 deaths and dozens injured (*Sydney Morning Herald*, 2010). The Prime Minister of Australia at that time, Kevin Rudd, joined other world leaders in condemning the attacks and called for Israel to launch an investigation into the attacks (*The Age*, 2010). A fact-finding mission by the UN Human Rights Council found that Israeli forces had committed a series of violations under international law, including humanitarian and human rights law (Human Rights Council, 2010).

Al Qaeda

The 9/11 attacks in 2001 sent ripples of fear across the world. The attacks were largely attributed to the Al Qaeda terrorist group, formed in 1989 in response to the incursion of Soviet forces into Afghanistan. The group came to be headed by Osama bin Laden, in an hierarchical structure based in Afghanistan and initiating terrorist attacks against western targets across the world (Mishal and Rosenthal, 2005). Debate flourishes in the literature as to what exactly Al Qaeda is. In a 2003 paper, Hoffman posed a number of questions regarding Al Qaeda:

> Is it a monolithic worldwide terrorist organisation with an identifiable hierarchical command; has it become a franchise operation with likeminded local representatives independently advancing the parent organisation's goals?; is it a concept, a virus, an army or an ideology?
>
> (p. 4)

It is likely that the same questions are being asked in 2014, as Al Qaeda is still a relatively secret organisation with branches and sub-groups in many countries. However, as more of its members are caught, questioned and killed – with the death of bin Laden himself in May 2011 – more information is beginning to emerge on its operations. Information is also being collated from modern forensic techniques and other information gained from the attacks it perpetrates throughout the world.

Regarding its operations, Mishal and Rosenthal (2005) suggest that Al Qaeda has two methods of operation, namely a hierarchical order and networks – a view which is relevant to the questions posed by Hoffman above. In other words, it is possibly 'both a hierarchal organisation and a franchise', with a 'fundamental aim to hurt America, Russia and Israel in an attempt to free the Arab world from Western domination' (Raphael, cited in Mishal and Rosthenhal, 2005, p. 278).

It would seem that Al Qaeda initially had a hierarchical structure at its origin in Afghanistan but then, post-Afghanistan, moved to a network approach, with 'transnational features and a willingness of Osama to fight on behalf of multiple causes with similar objectives' (Mishal and Rosenthal, 2005, p. 280). According to these authors, an example of this is the goal of Jemaah Islamiyah (JI), an extremist organisation with the primary aim of creating a pan-Islamic state in South East Asia (Mishal and Rosenthal, 2005). JI was accused of involvement in the 2002 Bali bombings and was said to have strong links to Al Qaeda.

Bio-terrorism

As in most western countries, Australian intelligence agencies and policy-makers have become increasingly concerned by the potential threat of terrorist attacks employing non-conventional weapons and methods. Much of the focus on this 'new' terrorism has highlighted the potential use of weapons of mass destruction (WMD), such as chemical, biological, radiological or nuclear (CBRN) weapons, against civilian targets. The Australian Minister for Foreign Affairs and Trade at the time of the Bali bombings, Alexander Downer, described the threat from WMD terrorism as the 'ultimate horror' (Downer, 2002, p. 8).

Biological weapons are not a new phenomenon; the technology to produce these agents has been available to terrorists for a number of years. Bio-terrorism appeals to terrorists as the organisms are small, are easy to carry and can produce mass fear and disarray in the targeted countries. This fear and disarray was noticeable in America following the intentional release of anthrax spores in 2001 (Brookmeyer and Blades, 2003). The Soviet Union reportedly stockpiled biological agents during the Cold War (Dattwyler, 2004), and such agents have already been used by the Aum Shinrikyo sect in Japan (Olson, 2009). Saddam Hussein also used chemical weapons to kill approximately 5,000 civilian victims in 1998 (Dattwyler, 2004) and more recently, in September 2013, a UN delegation accused the Syrian regime of using chemical weapons against civilians including children, against international law (UN Report, 2013).

Bio-terrorism protection measures were singled out by the Clinton administration in 1995 for special funding and attention. The administration set up training programs for bio-terrorism first responders, stockpiled vaccines and took measures to improve communication networks (Jones, 2005). By 2002 the Bush administration had spent $1.1 billion to protect citizens from terrorist attacks through measures such as the protection of food and water supplies (Jones, 2005). The intentional release of agents designed to induce a communicable disease in a country's population is being discussed and planned for by many governments and health departments across the world. Anthrax is not the only biological threat; from as early as 2003, EEC health departments were discussing the need for early recognition of a range of diseases which could be deliberately used by terrorists as weapons, such as anthrax, plague, botulism and the Ebola virus (Fadda and Paola, 2003).

Economic terrorism

In the days following 9/11, Osama bin Laden commented that 'every dollar of al-Qaida defeated a million dollars by the permission of Allah, besides the loss of a huge number of jobs' (cited in Whyte, 2007). The cost of terrorism, in terms of the loss of life, injury and effects on victims' family and friends, is immeasurable. As discussed, the objectives of terrorism are usually considered to kill, injure or instil fear. However, economic terrorism describes strategies which are specifically designed to disrupt a country's economy. As a result of the Bali bombing, a large number of tourists stayed away from the island due to security concerns, which resulted in a rise in unemployment levels and a fall of 25 per cent in household income levels across the island. Eight months after the bombing, some industries were reporting 80 per cent declines in turnover (Hospitality Net Industry News, 2005). It is unclear, however, if these effects on the Balinese economy were direct objectives of the attack.

Egyptian terrorists' targeting and bombing of foreign tourists in the early 1980s can be seen as a blueprint for such terrorist acts. These produced similar results to those found in Bali, in that tourists stayed away in large numbers and the country's economy was adversely affected (Cetron, 1994). It is thought that the 9/11 attacks in America were designed to disrupt the US economy as well as the economies of other western countries. Terrorists are aware that attacks of such magnitude are widely reported by the world's media, especially when tourists or civilians of other nations are killed or injured, and that this will lead to a large decline in tourism earnings. There are therefore both direct and indirect costs to the nations involved.

Apart from the direct costs of loss of life and property damage, terrorist attacks unsettle the target country's economy, resulting in slower economic growth and capital losses on stock markets (Nanto, 2004). They also push governments across the world to protect citizens by injecting many millions of dollars into counter-terrorism measures. This results in budget cuts for other important projects, as was demonstrated in Australia when the federal government invested large sums in counterterrorism measures and cut state budgets following both the 9/11 and Bali attacks. Overall, the 9/11 attacks were reported to have weakened an already slow world economy, with projected growth of GDP in 185 countries across the world reaching 1.95 per cent instead of the previously forecast 3.1 per cent (Nanto, 2004).

The future of terrorism and terrorist organisations

Paragraph 4 of the UN Security Council Resolution 1373, Sept 2001, notes with concern 'the close connections between international terrorism and illicit drugs, money laundering, illegal arms trafficking and illegal movement' (United Nations Security Council, 2001, p. 3). As discussed, terrorism has evolved and adapted over many hundreds of years and is likely to continue to do so. In a 1994 review of the future face of terrorism, Cetron (1994) predicted that the most ominous trend in terrorism would be related to technology. In this paper he postulated that biological or chemical weapons, and the technology that goes with them, will eventually be available to terrorist groups, organised crime and even individuals. He further suggested that these groups would be joined by fanatical single-issue terrorist groups and groups which are motivated by religious fervour, coining the phrase 'super terrorism' to describe them. For the most part, Cetron's predictions have come true, with the rise of the modern-day terrorist who uses technology and criminal activity to further their cause.

Terrorists have also used the technique of laundering the proceeds of their crimes to finance their activities. Steps have been taken by countries such as America and Australia to reduce this illegal activity by investing large sums of money in counterterrorism efforts. Since 1999, money-laundering strategies have been developed annually in the US, and following 9/11 staff training was increased to ensure that staff in banks and other financial organisations were aware of and able to stop terrorist money-laundering (McCullogh and Pickering, 2005). It has been argued by others that this type of financial hypervigilance has pushed terrorist groups to increase their criminal activities (Hutchinson and O'Malley, 2007). Others have suggested that due to increased security, organisations launder their money through other countries where the financial and legal systems are not quite so vigilant, such as Saudi Arabia (Mishal and Rosenthal, 2005).

The context of the Bali study – terrorist attacks in Indonesia

Indonesia is a former Dutch and Japanese colony which gained independence in 1958. It is the world's largest archipelago, consisting of over 17,500 islands spread over an arc of 3,000 miles. The country is divided into 33 provinces with a population of over 200 million (Hoey, 2003). The Bali attacks of 2002 and 2005 have been widely discussed in the popular press, but Indonesia has experienced other terrorist attacks, such as those in Aceh. Aceh has been a province of Indonesia since its independence in 1949 and since the 1950s there has been a general state of unrest in the province, related to the fight for independence. The Free Aceh movement has continued to mount terrorist attacks on civilian targets and the Indonesian police and military. The Indonesian military frequently retaliates with counterinsurgency tactics which have been criticised as 'heavy handed reprisals' (Schulze, 2004, p. 74). In addition to the attacks on Bali, other incidents have occurred in the nation's capital, Jakarta, with the attacks blamed on Islamic militants.

The Bali bombings and their impact

On 12 October 2002, two bombs exploded on Legian Street in Kuta. In a report prepared by Yayasan IDEP (2003) the sequence of events is catalogued, using local and international eyewitness accounts. The first bomb was detonated at 11.08 pm in Paddy's bar and café. Many people ran out of the Sari club, another popular nightclub opposite Paddy's bar, to see what the noise was. Just three minutes later a second, much larger, suicide bomb was detonated in a large white panel van parked outside the Sari club. The second bomb was clearly aimed at the tourists inside and outside the club, and resulted in a large fire which quickly engulfed the flimsy bamboo, wood and straw-built club. As a result of the fire the electricity supply was destroyed, resulting in the entire area's lighting system failing. The only available light came from the inferno surrounding Paddy's bar and the Sari club across an area of approximately 200 metres. Locally the area became known as 'ground zero' (Yayasan IDEP, 2003). This comparison with 9/11 continues in Australia, with the attacks being referred to as 'Australia's September 11' (Australian Federal Police, 2002).

The victims

The majority of deaths occurred in the nightclub, the bar and surrounding streets. The Sari nightclub and Paddy's bar had a long tradition of being popular night-time venues for young tourists to visit. On the night of 12 October 2002 many hundreds of international tourists were inside the club and bar. Tourists, staff and those inside and outside the clubs and restaurants of Legian Street became terrorist targets and many were killed or injured (see Table 1.1). In 2003, a national workshop entitled 'Lessons learnt from the health sector response to the Bali bomb blast' (World Health Organization, 2003) reported that the large number of burns patients and those with other injuries, totalling 300 in all, over-whelmed the available health services despite a tremendous response from all the personnel involved. A third bomb, which was the subject of less reporting, was detonated close to the American, Australian and Japanese embassies in the capi-tal, Denpasar, 13 minutes after the Kuta bombs (Yayasan IDEP, 2003). This bomb only slightly damaged the fences surrounding the buildings and no loss of life was reported. The three bombs were unexpected: Bali had previously been a peaceful and safe destination for tourists, expatriates and residents. Table 1.1 provides an overview of the victims and damage to property as recorded in the Yayasan IDEP (2003) report.

Table 1.1 Official total of blast victims and damage

Victims	Deceased	Injured	Total	Notes
Indonesian	37	205	242	
Australian	91	120	285	
Other nationalities	74*	Combined		*Victims included 20 other nationalities
Totals	**202**	**325**	**527**	
Damaged/Destroyed	Destroyed	Damaged		
Buildings	53	400		
Cars	18			
Motorcycles	32			

Source: Yayasan IDEP, 2003

The wider effects of the bombing

If, as suggested by Susser and Susser (2002), the primary target of terrorism is a country's psychological well-being, these attacks met their objective. In Bali the effects were perhaps best summed up by a local male resident, who was heard at the time to say: 'we are all dead now' (Brace, 2003, p. 28). Apart from the phys-ical and psychological damage experienced by the victims of and witnesses to the disaster, the bombings deeply affected the Balinese community and its belief systems. Indonesia is a predominately Muslim country, while Bali is a mainly Hindu enclave (Solomon, 2002). Many of the Balinese residents considered the bomb to have disrupted the 'natural balance' which is traditionally respected in Balinese Hindu culture (Sedana, 2005). To the Balinese Hindu people, life revolves around this natural balance between Bali's material and spiritual worlds. That harmony is termed *Tri Hita Karana*, a harmony between heaven, humans and the earth.

To the Balinese, the bombings totally disrupted this natural harmony; they deeply unsettled the population, who believed that disgruntled gods and evil spirits had been at work (Solomon, 2002). In mid-November 2002, in an effort to restore the balance, the local priests held a *Tawar Agung Pamarisudha Karipubhaya* ceremony at the bomb sites and the local beach. The Balinese believed that by cleansing the site with holy water and making offerings, harmony and balance would be regained in the world and in Bali (YKIP, 2007). Unfortunately, it would take more than this lovely, peaceful ceremony for the victims of all levels to recover their social, psychological and physical harmony.

The island of Bali

Bali is one of the smallest islands in the Indonesian archipelago, just 5,632 square kilometres in size (Figure 1.1). The island is densely populated and has approximately three million inhabitants, most of whom reside in the southern coastal areas. As noted, 90 per cent of Balinese follow the Hindu religion, setting the island apart from the rest of Indonesia, where the predominant religion is Muslim (Eiseman, 2005).

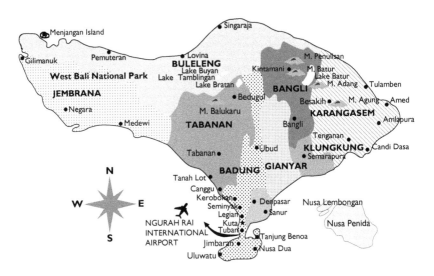

Figure 1.1 Map of Bali

Bali has been described as 'the Island of the Gods', as found in this translation of an inscription in the Purana Sada Temple of Kapal Traditional Village:

> It is said that when the continents and various island had been created on earth, Ida Sang Hyang Widhi/Bathara Pasupati (God), summoned the Gods to gather together on top of Mount Mahameru. Then Sang Hyang Pasupati uttered to the nine Gods occupying the nine directions, to the six Gods (Sad Winayaka), to the group four Gods (Catur Dewa), to God Rsis, to God Dragon, Gods from Trinayaka group and to Gods in the universe, to make a new island known as Bali.
>
> (History of Bali, 2010)

Local migration

Indonesia is densely inhabited, with an imbalance in population distribution among the islands: Java and Bali are more heavily populated. To help alleviate this problem, successive Indonesian governments have continued a voluntary (and sometimes involuntary) policy initiated by the Dutch in 1905 to resettle Indonesians from the heavily populated areas to the outer island provinces such as Northern Sumatra, Sulawesi and Kalimantan (Tirtosudarmo, 2009, p. 4). This social experiment was later supported by the central government of President Suharto, as well as outside interests such as large oil companies and the World Bank. Financial support from outside interests ceased in the 1980s due to the criticism which surfaced because of the wide-reaching socio-economic effects of the scheme. For many, the promise of paradise in the outer islands didn't materialise; the schemes (and some of the people administering them) were accused of mismanagement and corruption. Due to increasing regional autonomy, the practice of forced migration has greatly reduced (Hoey, 2003).

Throughout this period Bali continued to thrive economically, with increasing arrivals of international and domestic tourists from the late 1960s onwards. As a consequence, migrants began to flock to Bali in search of work. In 2007 there were 1,500 non-Indonesians working in tourism-related industries and 100,000 Indonesians from regions outside of Bali employed in the small trade sectors such as sales, handicraft, farming and fishing industries (Turker, 2007). This mass input of people produced a change in the demographics of Bali, from mainly Balinese Hindus to a population of more than three million people described as multi-ethnic and multi-religious (Bali guide, n.d.). Tensions do arise from time to time between residents and new migrants. In the early part of 1998 there were a series of riots across Indonesia, including in Bali, mainly in the form of attacks against Chinese-owned businesses, as simmering social unrest and bad feeling against migrant workers grew (United Nations High Commissioner for Refugees [UNHCR], 1998). Such tensions were heightened following the bombings in 2002 as the locals became suspicious of outsiders or non-Balinese (personal communication, 15 January 2008).

Farming and tourism

Historically, subsistence farming was the primary means of earning a living in Bali (Suartika, 2005). This was mainly in the form of wet rice propagation and fruit and vegetable farming. For centuries the farmers used a land cultivation method known as *sabak*, a traditional and eco-friendly irrigation system which does not put excess demands on the land and is sustainable. With rapidly expanding tourist need for accommodation, shops and recreation areas, as much as 1,000 hectares of paddy fields are taken over by developers each year. As a result there is a significantly reduced need for and use of the traditional irrigation system, less land available for farming and fewer young people willing or available to carry out the traditional ownership and farming tasks (Sutawan, 2005).

There is growing discussion within Bali on the need to take action on the effects of tourism on the landscape and people, with Suartika summing up the crisis in the title and subject matter of his thesis, 'Vanishing paradise: Planning and conflict in Bali' (2005), in which he argues that Bali, its culture and its traditional way of life is under attack from a number of factors which include the previously discussed tourism development, the continued migration of workers from outside Bali and under-regulated development (Suartika, 2005). In an effort to avert the effects of under-regulated development and migration, there is a move towards eco-tourism in Bali. A 2007 report recognised the problems inherent in mass tourism and recommended a need to promote cultural tourism in Bali which includes 'an integral unit of ecosystem, spatial arrangement, physical environment and Balinese culture' (Ashrama *et al*, 2007, p. 125), a concept which is in keeping with the ideals of the previously discussed spiritual concept of *Tri Hita Kirana*.

Tourism gained momentum in Bali from the mid to late 1980s, reaching a peak of one million visitors per year in the late 1990s. Around 1,000 hotels were developed to meet demand, based around the popular tourist hubs of Sanur, Nusa Dua, Kuta and Ubud (United Nations Development Programme Fund, 2003, p. 6). Tourism eventually became Indonesia's second-largest foreign exchange earner (after gas and oil). According to a World Bank Report in 2003, Bali had developed a healthy economy with a poverty rate of only 4 per cent – a stark contrast with the rate of 16 per cent for the rest of Indonesia (United Nations Development Programme Fund, 2003, p. 7).

Tourists in Bali include direct arrivals from overseas and indirect arrivals from other parts of Indonesia. The island's dependence on the tourism industry was demonstrated by the economic effects of the Bali bombings in 2002. Tourists became too frightened to holiday in Bali and stayed away. Suartika (2005) reports the number of tourists entering Bali dropped to less than a third of the usual levels in the months following the 2002 bombing, resulting in tourist facilities and businesses closing down and tens of thousands of people being made redundant. The resultant economic and social effect was devastating.

Suartika argues this was a prime example of how previous decades of tourism growth had made Bali 'economically and otherwise wholly dependent on tourism' (Suartika, 2005, p. 3).

Socio-economic impact of the bombing

The socio-economic effect of the bombing was widespread and not limited to the hotel and tourist industry. Smaller related areas such as the art and handicraft industries, taxi drivers, market traders, t-shirt manufacturers and beach vendors were all affected. Overall unemployment levels rose, income levels fell by 43 per cent across the island and, eight months after the bombing, some industries were reporting a decline in turnover of 80 per cent. As a result of this, many families throughout the island were living below the poverty line (World Bank, 2003, p. 7).

The tourists return

International experience of terrorist attacks suggests that their effects on tourism are temporary. With time and effort directed at increasing tourist confidence, tourists do eventually return (Maditinos and Vassiliadis, 2008). In Bali, measures such as a visibly increased security presence and the swift capture of the bombers resulted in a gradual return of tourists, and by 2005 tourist arrivals totalled 5,002,101. They continued to increase in the following years, with tourist arrivals to Indonesia totalling 6.42 million in 2008, an increase of 13.24 per cent on the previous year (Tourism Indonesia, 2009). Total tourist arrivals in Indonesia in the first quarter of 2012 stood at 1.9 million, an increase of 11.01 per cent on 1.71 million the previous year (*The Bali Times*, 2012).

Summary

The reality is that terrorist attacks are likely to continue to occur and evolve. As terrorist organisations evolve and change their tactics, so too do methods of detection. Ordinary, non-combatant citizens innocently going about their daily lives will likely continue to be the targets of attack. History has demonstrated that terrorist organisations will continue to thrive despite the might of whatever defence mechanisms are used in response, whether a war on terror or imprisonment of those merely suspected of being terrorists.

Chapter 2 catalogues the methodological approaches and study design used in the current study.

Notes

1 The Madrid train bombings were a series of co-ordinated bombings on the morning commuter train system in Madrid, Spain on 11 March 2004 which killed 191 people and wounded 1,800.

2 The 2008 Mumbai attacks involved more than ten co-ordinated shooting and bombing attacks across Mumbai. The attacks were spread over three days in November and resulted in the deaths of 173 people and the wounding of 308.

3 Co-ordinated terrorist bombings on the London underground and bus service on 7 July 2005 (also known as 7/7) in which 52 commuters were killed and over 700 wounded.

References

The Age (2010, 1 June). Global condemnation of Israeli raid. Retrieved 20 May 2014 from http://www.theage.com.au/world/global-condemnation-of-israeli-raid-20100531-wrag.html

Ashrama, B., Pitana, I. G., and Windia, W. (2007). Bali is Bali forever. Sustainability in the framework of Tri Hita Karana. Bali Travel News and P.T Post, pp. 186–193.

Australian Federal Police (2002). Bali Bombings 2002. Retrieved 20 May 2014 from http://www.afp.gov.au/international/operations/previous

Australia's emergency response to the Bali bombings (2005). The Australian Journal of Emergency Management, 20(4), 33. Retrieved 20 May 2014 from http://www.ag.gov.au/www/emaweb/rwpattach.nsf/VAP/%2899292794923AE8E7CBABC6FB71541EE1%29~Australia%27s+Emergency+Response+to+the+Bali+Bombings.pdf/$file/Australia%27s+Emergency+Response+to+the+Bali+Bombings.pdf

Bali Guide (n.d.) Introduction to Bali. Retrieved 20 May 2014 from http://www.baliguide.com/geography.html

The Bali Times (2012, 9 May). Tourist numbers continue to rise. The Bali Times. Retrieved 10 April 2014 from www.thebalitimes.com/2012/05/09/tourist-numbers-continue-to-rise/

BBC News (2009, 8 March). Baghdad police attack 'kills 28'. Retrieved 20 May 2014 from http://news.bbc.co.uk/2/hi/7930958.stm

BBC News. (2011, 18 December). Last US troops withdraw from Iraq. Retrieved 20 May 2014 from http://www.bbc.co.uk/news/world-middle-east-16234723.

Bhattacharji, P. (2008). Liberation Tigers of Tamil Elam (aka Tamil Tigers) (Sri Lanka, separatists). Council on Foreign Relations. Retrieved 20 May 2014 from http://www.cfr.org/publications

Brace, M. (2003). The road back to Bali. Geographical, 75(10), 26–34.

Brookmeyer, R., and Blades, N. (2003). Statistical models and bioterrorism: Application to the US anthrax outbreak. Journal of the American Statistical Association, 98(464), 781–788.

Cetron, M. J. (1994). The future face of terrorism. The Futuris, 28(6), 1–10.

Chevigney, B. (2007). UNICEF Representative in Somalia assesses impact of conflict on children and families. Retrieved 20 May 2014 from http://www.unicef.org/infobycountry/somalia_38023.html

Chulov, M. (2010, 12 May). Allawai warns of sectarian war. The Sydney Morning Herald. Retrieved 20 May 2014 from http://www.smh.com.au/world/allawi-warns-of-sectarian-war-20100511-uuba.html

Cooper, H. (2014). Kurdish forces in Iraq secure Kirkuk as ISIS militants continue their push toward Baghdad. ABC News. Retrieved 20 May 2014 from http://www.abc.net.au/news/2014-06-12/kirkuk-secured-as-isis-insurgents-close-in-on-baghdad/5520146

Cooper, H., Landler, M., and Rubin, A. J. (2014, 7 August). Obama allows limited airstrikes on ISIS. New York Times. Retrieved 20 May 2014 from http://www.nytimes.com/

2014/08/08/world/middleeast/obama-weighs-military-strikes-to-aid-trapped-iraqis-officials-say.html?_r=0

Dattwyler, R. J. (2004). Community-acquired pneumonia in the age of terrorism. *Pulmonary Medicine, 12*(3), 240–249.

De Young, K. (2009, 28 February). Obama sets timetable for Iraq. *Washington Post.* Retrieved 20 May 2014 from http://www.washingtonpost.com/wpdyn/content/article/2009/02/27/AR2009022700566.html

DeLisi, L. E., Maurizio, A., Yost, M., Papparozzi, C. F., Fulchino, C., Katz, C. L., Altesman, J., Biel, M., Lee, J., and Stevens, P. (2003). A survey of New Yorkers after the Sept. 11, 2001 terrorist attacks. *American Journal of Psychiatry, 160*(4), 780–783.

Downer, A. (2002, 17 September). Iraq: Weapons of mass destruction. Statement to the Australian Parliament.

Dougall, A. L., Hayward, M. C., and Baum, A. (2005). Media exposure to bioterrorism: stress and the anthrax attacks. *Psychiatry: Interpersonal and Biological processes, 68*(1), 28–42.

The Economist (2014, 3 May). Iraq's election: Alas it may make little difference. The incumbent prime minister holds on like grim death. Retrieved 20 May 2014 from http://www.economist.com/news/middle-east-and-africa/21601576-incumbent-prime-minister-holds-grim-death-alas-it-may-make-little

Eiseman, F. (2005). *Bali, sekala and niskala. Essays on religion, ritual and art.* Hong Kong: Periplus Editions Ltd.

Fadda, G., and Paola, C. (2003). Risks and actions against bio-terrorism in Europe. *The European Journal of Public Health, 13*(2), 1–8.

Galbraith, P. (2006). *The end of Iraq: How American incompetence created a war without end.* New York: Simon and Schuster.

Gearson, J. (2002). The nature of modern terrorism. *The Political Quarterly, 73,* 7–24.

Goodhand, J., Klem, B., and Sørbø, G. (2011). *Pawns of peace: Evaluation of Norwegian peace efforts in Sri Lanka, 1997–2009.* Report commissioned by Norad Evaluation Department, Report 5/2011, Copenhagen.

Hassan, S. R. (2014). Taliban gunmen attack Karachi airport academy in second assault. *Reuters.* Retrieved 20 May 2014 from http://www.reuters.com/article/2014/06/10/us-pakistan-army-idUSKBN0EL09I20140610

Hirsch, M. L. and Wolfe, L. (2012). Women under siege profile: Democratic Republic of Congo. Retrieved 15 July 2014 from http://www.womenundersiegeproject.org/conflicts/profile/democratic-republic-of-congo

History of Bali. (2010). Retrieved 20 May 2014 from http://www.2indonesia.com/history.htm

Hoey, B. A. (2003). Nationalism in Indonesia: Building imagined and intentional communities through transmigration. *University of Michigan Ethnology, 42*(2), 109–126.

Hoffman, B. (2003). *Al Qaeda, trends in terrorism, and future potentialities: An assessment.* Retrieved 20 May 2014 from http://www.rand.org/pubs/papers/P8078/P8078.pdf

Holmes, J. (2009, October 6). One-third of Gaza dead, injured are children. *ABC News.* Retrieved 20 May 2014 from http://abcnews.go.com/International/wireStory?id=6609055

Hospitality Net Industry News (2005). *First update on hotel performance in Bali since the October attacks: Deloitte reports.* Retrieved 20 May 2014 from http://www.hospitalitynet.org/news/4025411.search?query=balines%20economy%20delotte%2c%202005

Human Rights Council (2010). *Report of the international fact-finding mission to investigate violations of international law, including international humanitarian and human rights law, resulting from the Israeli attacks on the flotilla of ships carrying humanitarian assistance.* United Nations General Assembly. A/HRC/15/21, 1–66.

Hutchinson, S., and O'Malley, P. (2007). A crime–terror nexus? Thinking on some of the links between terrorism and criminality. *Studies in Conflict and Terrorism, 30*(12), 1095–1107.

Institute for Economics and Peace (IEP). (2012). *Global terrorism index: Capturing the impact of terrorism for the last decade.* Retrieved 20 May 2014 from http://www.visionofhumanity.org/sites/default/files/2012_Global_Terrorism_Index_Report.pdf

Israel Ministry of Foreign Affairs (2014). *Victims of Palestinian violence and terrorism since September 2000.* Retrieved 20 May 2014 from http://www.mfa.gov.il/mfa/foreignpolicy/terrorism/palestinian/pages/victims%20of%20palestinian%20violence%20and%20terrorism%20sinc.aspx

Jerard, J., Astuti, F., and Feisal, M. (2009, July). *Bombing of the JW Marriot and Ritz Carlton, Jakarta.* Retrieved 20 May 2014 from http://www.pvtr.org/pdf/GlobalAnalysis/BombingOfTheJWMarriott&RitzCarltonJakartaReport.pdf

Jones, D. (2005). Structure of bio-terrorism preparedness in the UK and the US: Responses to 9/11 and the anthrax attacks. *British Journal of Politics and Human Relations, 7*(3), 340–352.

Kaplan, E. H., Mintz, A., and Mishal, S. (2006). Tactical prevention of suicide bombings in Israel. *Interfaces, 36*(6), 553–561.

Maditinos, Z., and Vassiliadis, C. (2008). *Crisis and disasters in tourism industry: Happen locally – affect globally,* 67–76. Retrieved 20 May 2014 from http://mibes.teilar.gr/e-books/2008/maditinos_vasiliadis%2067-76.pdf

McCullogh, J., and Pickering, S. (2005). Suppressing the financing of terrorism: Proliferating state crime, eroding censure and extending neo-colonialism. *British Journal of Criminology, 45,* 470–486.

Mahmoud, M. (2010, 18 June). Car bomb in Iraq's restive north kills 7, wounds 61. *Reuters.* Retrieved 20 May 2014 from http://www.reuters.com/article/idUSTRE65H1W520100618

Michael, G., and Scolnick, J. (2006). The strategic limits of suicide terrorism in Iraq. *Small Wars and Insurgencies, 17*(2), 113–125.

Mielniezuk, M. (2009, July 30). Two officers killed in Mallorca car blast. *The Independent.* Retrieved 20 May 2014 from http://www.independent.co.uk/news/world/europe/two-police-killed-in-mallorca-blast-1764884.html

Miller, L. (2004). Psychotherapeutic interventions for survivors of terrorism. American Journal of Psychotherapy, *58*(1), 1–16.

Mishal, S., and Rosenthal, M. (2005). Al Qaeda as a dune organisation: Toward a typology of Islamic terrorist organisations. *Studies in Conflict and Terrorism, 28*(4), 275–293.

Mitchell, J. A. (2006). Soldier girl? Not every Tamil teen wants to be a Tiger. *The Humanist, 66*(5), 16–18. Retrieved 20 May 2014 from http://www.thehumanist.org/humanist/articles/Mitchell-SeptOct06.pdf

Moghadam, A. (2003). Palestinian suicide terrorism in the second Intifada: Motivations and organisational aspects. *Studies in Conflict and Terrorism, 26*(2), 65–92.

Nanto, K. D. (2004). *9/11 terrorism: Global economic costs.* CRS Report for Congress. Congressional Research Service. Retrieved 20 May 2014 from http://digital.library.unt.edu/ark:/67531/metacrs7725

Obama, B. (2014, May). *Statement by the President on Afghanistan*. Retrieved 20 May 2014 from http://www.whitehouse.gov/the-press-office/2014/05/27/statement-president-afghanistan

Olson, K. B. (2009). Aum Shinrikyo (1999) Once and future threat. *Journal of Emerging Infectious Diseases, 5*(4): 513–516.

Oxfam (2008). *The Gaza Strip: A humanitarian implosion*. Retrieved 20 May 2014 from http://www.oxfam.org.uk/resources/policy/conflict_disasters/gaza_implosion.html

Pape, R. A. (2003). The strategic logic of suicide terrorism. *The American Political Science Review, 97*(3), 343–347.

Pastor, L. H. (2004). Countering the psychological consequences of suicide terrorism. *Psychiatric Annals, 34*(9), 701–707.

Peace Direct. (2013, January). *Afghanistan: Conflict profile*. Retrieved 20 May 2014 from http://www.insightonconflict.org/conflicts/afghanistan/conflict-profile/

Powell, C. (2004). Did terrorism sway Spain's election? *Current History, 103*(676), 376–377.

Ramasubramanian, R. (2004). Suicide terrorism in Sri Lanka. *Institute of Peace and Conflict Studies Research Paper, 5*(1), 1–30. Retrieved 20 May 2014 from www.ipcs.org

Rolston, B., and Gilmartin, M. (2000). *Unfinished business: State killings and the quest for truth*. Belfast: Beyond the Pale Publications.

Rule of Law in Armed Conflicts (RULAC) Project (2014). *Democratic Republic of Congo – Current conflicts*. Retrieved 20 May 2014 from http://www.geneva-academy.ch/RULAC/current_conflict.php?id_state=178)

Schulze, K. E. (2004). The free Aceh movement (GAM): Anatomy of a separatist organisation. *Policy Studies, 2*, 1–76.

Sedana, I. N. (2005). Theatre in a time of terrorism: Renewing natural harmony after the Bali bombing via Wayang Kontemporer. *Asian Theatre Journal, 22*(11), 73–87.

Shah, A. (2010). *The Democratic Republic of Congo*. Retrieved 20 May 2014 from http://www.globalissues.org/article/87/the-democratic-republic-of-congo

Shekhar, M. (2009). Crisis management – a case study on Mumbai terrorist attack. *European Journal of Scientific Research, 27*(93), 358–371.

Sheppard, B. (2009). *The psychology of strategic terrorism: Public and governmental responses to attack*. Oxon: Routledge.

Solomon, J. (2002, 23 December). In wake of terror, Balinese offer goats, geese to angry Gods – bombing priests busy dispatching lost souls; cabbie's fare disappears. *Wall Street Journal*, pp. 1–4.

Somalia Civil War (n.d.) Retrieved 15 Jul 2014 from http://www.globalsecurity.org/military/world/war/somalia.htm

Suartika, G. A. (2005). *Vanishing paradise: Planning and conflict in Bali*. (Unpublished doctoral dissertation). University of New South Wales, Sydney, Australia. Retrieved 20 May 2014 from www.unsw.edu.au

Susser, E., and Susser, M. (2002). The aftermath of September 11: What's an epidemiologist to do? *International Journal of Epidemiology, 31*, 719–721.

Sutawan, N. (2005, November). *Tri Hita Karana and Subak. In search for alternative concept of sustainable irrigated rice culture*. Paper presented at the Network for Water and Ecosystem in Paddy Fields Conference, Tokyo, Japan. Retrieved 20 May 2014 from http://www.maff.go.jp/inwepf/documents/inaugural/sutawan-ppt.pdf

Sydney Morning Herald. (2010, 31 May). As many as 19 killed as flotilla stormed, says Israeli army. Retrieved 16 June 2011 from http://www.smh.com.au/world/as-many-as-19-killed-as-flotilla-stormed-says-israeli-army-20100531-wq8y.html

Tirtosudarmo, R. (2009). *Mobility and human development in Indonesia. Human Development Research Paper, 2009/19*. (United Nations Development Programme Research Paper), 1–73. Retrieved 20 May 2014 from http://hdr.undp.org/en/reports/global/hdr2009/papers/HDRP_2009_19.pdf

Tourism Indonesia (2009, 17 February). *National tourism arrivals up 13.24% in 2008*. Retrieved 20 May 2014 from http://www.tourismindonesia.com/2009/02/national-tourism-arrivals-up-1324-in.html

Tripp, A. M. (2004). The changing face of authoritarianism in Africa today. *Africa Today, 50*(3), 1–25.

Turker, S. (2007). Migration and tourism – Impact of migrant workers on tourism in Bali. Tourism and migration – Two windows into globalization. *Contours, 17*(2), 1–2.

UN Report. (2013). *UN Mission to investigate allegations of the use of chemical weapons in the Syrian Arab Republic*. Retrieved 20 May 2014 from http://www.un.org/disarmament/content/slideshow/Secretary_General_Report_of_CW_Investigation.pdf

UN Media Report. (2014, 7 August). *UN calls for urgent response to help thousands in Northern Iraq displaced by militants advance and ISIL*. Retrieved 20 May 2014 from http://www.un.org/apps/news/story.asp?NewsID=48439#.U–DiKOQ_IX

UN News Centre (2014, 13 June). *Afghanistan and the United Nations*. Retrieved 20 May 2014 from http://www.un.org/News/dh/latest/afghan/un-afghan-history.shtml

UN Secretary-General Report. (2013, 15 May). Democratic Republic of the Congo. Retrieved 20 May 2014 from http://childrenandarmedconflict.un.org/countries/democratic-republic-of-the-congo/

United Nations Assistance Mission for Iraq. (2006). *Human rights report*. Retrieved 20 May 2014 from http://unami.unmissions.org/LinkClick.aspx?fileticket=A6XvzkE9enU%3D&tabid=3174&language=en-US

United Nations Assistance Mission in Afghanistan. (2014, 9 Feb). *U.N. Assistance Mission in Afghanistan (UNAMA) Protection of Civilians in Armed Conflict 2013 Annual Report*. Retrieved 20 May 2014 from http://unama.unmissions.org/LinkClick.aspx?fileticket=OhsZ29Dgeyw%3D&tabid=12254&mid=15756&language=en-US press release july 2014

United Nations Development Programme Fund (2003). *Bali beyond the tragedy. Impact and challenges for tourism led development in Indonesia*. Jakarta, Indonesia: United Nations.

United Nations High Commissioner for Refugees (UNHCR) (1998). *Indonesia: Economic, social and political dimensions of the current crisis*. Retrieved 20 May 2014 from http://www.unhcr.org/refworld/docid/3ae6a6c50.html

United Nations Office for the Coordination of Humanitarian Affairs (UNOCHA). (2007, August 9). *Israeli–Palestinian casualties since 2000 – key trends*. Retrieved 20 May 2014 from http://www.ochaopt.org/

United Nations Security Council. (2001). *S/RES/1373*, 1–4. Retrieved 20 May 2014 from http://daccess-ods.un.org/TMP/7204300.16517639.html

USA Today. (2007, 15 February). Madrid bombing suspect denies guilt. Retrieved 20 May 2014 from http://www.usatoday.com/news/world/2007-02-15-madrid-terror-trial_x.htm

US State Department. (2003). *Patterns of global terrorism*, 1–6. Retrieved 20 May 2014 from http://www.state.gov/documents/organization/33889.pdf

Whyte, M. G. (2007). *The domestic economy and post 9/11 national security.* Unpublished report in partial fulfilment of graduation requirements. Maxwell Air Force Base, Alabama. Retrieved 20 May 2014 from https://www.afresearch.org/skins/rims/q_mod.../display.aspx

Wilson, N., and Thomson, G. (2005). The epidemiology of international terrorism involving fatal outcomes in developed countries (1994–2003). *European Journal of Epidemiology, 20*(5), 735–781.

Winkates, J. (2006). Suicide terrorism: Martyrdom for organisational objectives. *Journal of Third World Studies, 23*(1), 87–115.

World Bank. (2003). *Brief for the consultative group on Indonesia: Bali update: Confronting crisis: Impacts and response to the Bali tragedy*, 1–20. Retrieved 20 May 2014 from http://siteresources.worldbank.org/INTINDONESIA/Resources/CGI03/03-CGI/12CGI_BaliUpdate.pdf

World Health Organization (2003). Workshop on disaster management for the health sector in Indonesia, lessons learned from the Bali Bomb. Bali, Indonesia.

Yayasan IDEP. (2003). *The Bali bomb. A consolidated report on disaster management.* Ubud, Bali.

YKIP. (2007). YKIP's journey: The first five years. Bali, Indonesia: Annika Linden Foundation and Reset.

Chapter 2

An exploratory, qualitative case-study approach

This chapter explores how the current study was carried out and the research approach that was adopted, as well as offering a discussion of the work of the Psychosocial Working Group and how this was adapted for use in the current study.

Choosing a research approach – an exploratory qualitative approach

At the onset of any research, it is important to carefully consider the various research approaches available in order to match the approach with the aims and ethos of the study. In disaster studies, when there is a need to study feelings, experiences and meanings – particularly when the purpose of the research is to 'elicit understanding and not test [hypotheses]' (Poggenpoel and Myburgh, 2005, p. 304) – post-positivist qualitative research is a preferred methodology. This approach requires the researcher to employ 'a series of logically related steps, to believe in multiple perspectives rather than a single reality, and espouse multiple methods of data collection and analysis' (Creswell, 2007, p. 20). Therefore a qualitative research methodology in a real-world setting was chosen as the most appropriate method to gain knowledge and insight into the impacts of the 2002 Bali bombings. Further to this, it was hoped that the approach would then provide the opportunity to apply this knowledge to other disasters.

A qualitative case study of the Bali bombings in 2002

Qualitative research has evolved over many decades of research and an increase in its use has been reported in the literature (Daly *et al*, 2007; Lloyd-Jones, 2004). Consequently, qualitative research is now recognised as making a distinctive and important contribution to research and to disciplines such as health care, education and psychology (Capaldi and Proctor, 2005). The overarching aim of the core study in this book was to examine the multi-layered effects and forms of support received by victims of the 2002 Bali bombings in Indonesia and Australia. It was intended to give a 'voice' to the victims, as it was important that their story was heard in their own words. Therefore a case-study approach was the methodology of choice, as its main characteristics help bring the realities of the victim's experiences to the reader, and because it is a method which is now widely employed in social science research studies (Longden, 2001; Noor, 2008). The key components of a case-study approach appropriate to use in disaster studies are:

- First, it taps into the viewpoints of the participants (Tellis, 1997, p. 3).
- Second, it 'enables, and promotes' each participant an avenue to describe their experiences in their own words (Longden, 2001, p. 15).
- Third, it is the preferred methodology when there is a primary need to 'closely examine contemporary events' (Yin, 2003, p. 7).

Analysis using a psychosocial approach

The psychosocial approach to disaster mitigation is considered one of the most appropriate methods to assist populations affected by conflict and has been utilised many times after disasters such as 9/11 and the 2004 Boxing Day tsunami. A psychosocial approach underpins the analysis of the Bali situation outlined in this book. The primary reason for this recommendation is that the premise which underpins this approach is that communities whose resources are severely disrupted by terrorist attacks or disasters are able to help themselves, as they have a pool of pre-existing inherent resources which can be utilised in the aftermath of any type of major incident.

Also influencing this approach is the knowledge that within our everyday interactions we try to achieve a state of emotional, physical and social stability. It is this same state of stability which terrorist attacks and disasters challenge and disrupt. As a result, in emergencies there is a 'complex interplay between protection, threats and issues of mental health and psychosocial well-being' (Inter-Agency Standing Committee [IASC], 2006, p. 32). Therefore it seems appropriate that any approach to helping post-disaster should be aimed at assessing and supporting these elements and helping the affected population to help themselves.

The Psychosocial Working Group (PWG), established in 2000, has developed a framework for best practice in response to disasters. Within this framework they look beyond the usual focus on the mental health needs of individuals to the wider concept of the individual within their community and the loss of resources they experience, such as disruption to infrastructure, separation from their families and loss of income. As part of its attempt to better understand the disruptions experienced by individuals following a disaster, the group define psychosocial well-being as 'the social, cultural and psychological influences on wellbeing' (PWG, 2003, p. 1): the term 'psychosocial well-being' was used as humanitarian agencies and researchers began the quest to develop a conceptual framework which identified the complexities of needs individuals and communities experienced as a result of a disaster (PWG, 2003, p. 1).

To assist in this aim the PWG defined the psychosocial social aspects of well-being into three core domains, namely human capacity, social ecology and culture and values (PWG, 2003). The PWG viewed the categorisation of these domains as a way forward in helping to evaluate the trauma experienced by individuals and communities following disasters (PWG, 2003; Strang and Ager, 2001). These are the domains which the group consider to be challenged and disrupted by complex emergencies. Equally, as resources within these domains are disrupted, the PWG suggest there is 'a pool of resources' (PWG, 2003) within these domains which can be utilised by communities and individuals in their response to such emergencies. For example, human capacity may be engaged to promote social linkage, culture and values. Therefore individuals' and communities' adjustment and resilience to such events may be gauged by how effectively they exploit these resources (PWG, 2003).

These domains are highlighted in Figure 2.1. The semi-structured in-depth interviews in this study were based on this framework and helped gain valuable knowledge and insight into the multilayered effects of the bombing. Additionally, a pool of resources utilised by the two communities and individuals in the aftermath of the bombings was identified.

This framework is also useful for external support agencies such as the International Red Cross (IRC) and the World Health Organization (WHO) to plan their interventions when complex emergencies occur. During complex emergencies, well-meaning international aid is often mobilised by communities outside the countries affected, as was experienced following the 2004 Boxing Day tsunami. International communities will airlift support programmes, personnel and equipment to disaster areas as soon as possible after the disaster, but there is criticism of this approach as the agencies often attempt to 'restore' communities back to their pre-event state (Strang and Ager, 2001). This occurs because the agencies are naturally influenced by their own sets of social and cultural values from their

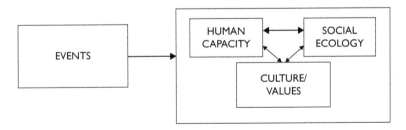

Figure 2.1 The three domains identified by the Psychosocial Working Group

Source: PWG, 2003 (used with permission)

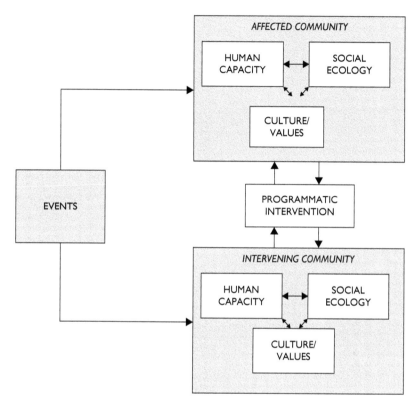

Figure 2.2 Programmatic intervention by the intervening community
Source: PWG, 2003 (used with permission)

country of origin, which fall within those same domains (Strang and Ager, 2001), as illustrated in Figure 2.2.

These values frequently conflict with the affected communities' core sets of values, particularly in developing countries, and can result in support programmes which are not culturally sensitive. Current intervention studies suggest it is preferable to assist countries affected by disaster to transform and utilise their own available resources. The long-term aim should be to allow a community to 'deploy its own resources and meet its challenges without the need for external (agency) support' (Strang and Ager, 2001, p. 6). This would seem appropriate, as individual countries are best placed to assess their own needs and available resources. With this background to the framework that underpinned the study, a matrix detailing the methodology used to address the aims of the study is presented in Table 2.1.

Table 2.1 Aims and associated methodology summaries

Aims	Methodology	Methods	Analysis
To investigate the multi-layered effects of the Bali bombings at the individual, family and community levels immediately following the bombing and in the intervening period.	Exploratory, qualitative, in-depth interviews with directly affected individuals (victims and family members) and indirectly affected individuals (friends, neighbours, community members).	Semi-structured interviews and open-ended questions.	Use of qualitative data analysis for emergence of themes.
To identify and examine the forms of post-attack support received by directly affected victims who were in the Sari club or Paddy's bar at the time of the attack, and their family members who became indirect victims of the attack.	Exploratory, qualitative, in-depth interviews with directly affected individuals (victims and family members) and indirectly affected individuals (friends, neighbours community members).	Semi-structured interviews and open-ended questions.	Use of qualitative data analysis for emergence of themes.
To document and examine the perceptions and comments of members of the Indonesian and Australian emergency response teams and community volunteers who assisted in the aftermath of the crisis.	Exploratory, qualitative, in-depth interviews with members of the emergency response team and community volunteers.	Interviews with members of the emergency response team and members of the volunteer community.	Use of qualitative data analysis for emergence of themes.
To systematically critique available literature on the multi-layered effects of terrorist attacks and the forms of post-attack support offered to victims and their families.	A comprehensive review of relevant literature relating to terrorist attacks and post-attack interventions.	A literature search of databases, e.g. ProQuest, PsycInfo, ScienceDirect, for peer-reviewed journal articles.	Literature summary and critical analysis of related literature.
To develop a framework of recommendations that may be used by professionals and non-professionals in the aftermath of a terrorist attack particularly when needing to choose appropriate and culturally relevant interventions.	Analysis of the participant interviews, researcher observations and collation of documentary data including media and related literature.	Participant interviews; literature review; frame analysis of media; relevant documentary data; reflective diary and researcher observations.	Assessment of the outcomes of the study and development of a possible framework.

The Bali field study – Bali research processes

Recruitment of supporting agency and research assistants

At 5,632 square kilometres, Bali is one of the smallest, and most densely popu-lated, of the 17,500 islands making up the Indonesian archipelago. It is situated eight degrees south of the equator, off the most easterly point of Java. The major-ity of the three million-plus people living in Bali (92 per cent in 2010) identify as Hindu (Malik, 2012). Following the 2002 bombing there was an influx of mon-etary donations to the island and a number of non-government agencies were established to support the affected Balinese population.

One of the organisations formed in 2002 is Yayasan Kemanusiaan Ibu Pertiwi (YKIP), which was formed to respond to the many needs of the Balinese victims in the initial stages of the crisis. Another, Yayasan Kids (YKIDS), was formed initially to fund the educational needs of children whose parents had been killed or injured in the bombing. In 2003 both organisations entered a memorandum of understanding agreement, with YKIP taking responsibility for fundraising and YKIDS the educational and outreach function. The YKIP–YKIDS partnership has subsequently grown into an organisation dedicated to serving the educational and health needs of those who live in Bali (YKIDS, 2002; YKIP, 2007). YKIP was approached to assist in the research process in Bali as it had initially been formed to support individuals and families who had been affected by the bombing. Importantly, YKIP's Chief Executive Officer agreed to support the study by assisting with access to participants selected from the directly affected population.

In addition, local research assistants were recruited; they assisted, as cultural interpreters, with individual interviews, questionnaire administration and tran-scription of the information gathered. The research assistants' roles were discussed early on in order to develop and build effective working relationships (Pitchforth and Van Teijlingen, 2005), which was essential to the research process.

Recruitment of participants

In total, 33 participants from Bali took part in the study (see Table 2.2). The participants were all residents of Bali and were classified as *primary-level victims* (10) of the 2002 bombing – that is, individuals who had maximum exposure to the terrorist bomb, such as those who were in the Sari nightclub or Paddy's bar at the time of the attacks; *secondary-level victims* (10), the family and friends of

Table 2.2 Participants recruited for interviews – Bali

Primary Victims	Secondary Victims	Third-Level Volunteers	Third-Level Professionals	Key Informants
6 Female	10 Female		3 Female	1 Female
4 Male		2 Male	4 Male	3 Male

the primary victims; *third-level victims* (7), the rescue, recovery and professional personnel who took part in the emergency response and were involved with the initial care of the victims; and the *key informant group* (4), people who had been indirectly affected by the bombings, such as tradespeople or residents of Bali. All participants were over 18 years of age.

Due to the sensitive nature of the research topic, and to reduce the risk of further distress to the participants, the following participants were excluded from the study:

- those who had been diagnosed with a mental health problem within the preceding 12 months;
- those who were receiving counselling or psychotherapeutic interventions for a mental health problem or had received such interventions within the preceding 12 months;
- those who were currently prescribed medication for a mental health problem.

Participants were identified by using purposive, volunteer, opportunistic and snowball techniques, using the contacts that had been established in the community. The roles of YKIP and YKIDS staff and a local doctor who worked part-time in private practice were centrally important in the sensitive recruitment of the participants. Indicative of this is that only three potential participants declined to take part in the current study.

Collecting the data

Once contact was made and an interview time agreed upon, the interviews were undertaken. Specifics for each victim group are detailed as follows. All of the interviews were audio-taped, after seeking permission to do so.

Primary-level victims (PLV) – this group consisted of six male participants and four female participants. All but one of the males had been working in the Sari club or Paddy's bar on the night of the bombing and had been directly affected by the bombing. The interviews were all conducted in the participants' homes in Kuta or Denpasar (which is situated approximately 15 kilometres from Kuta).

Secondary-level victims (SLV) – this group consisted of ten female participants whose family members had been either killed or injured in the bombing. They all were interviewed in their homes, which were in Denpasar, Kuta or the village of Tabanan.

Third-level victims (TLV) – this group consisted of nine participants, all volunteers and professionals who had provided support to the victims. Two were male volunteers who worked for the Red Cross at 'ground zero' (as the locals have termed the bombing sites in Legian Street and the morgue). Three were female volunteers supporting the families of victims. Four were male members of the medical profession, two who had worked as surgeons on the night and two who had worked as psychiatrists supporting victims or family members following the bombing.

Key informants – Three business owners were interviewed to gain further information regarding the economic effects on businesses in the Kuta area. A tailor, a hotel owner and a taxi driver, all of whose businesses had been adversely affected by the bombing, were interviewed. In addition, two key members of the Bali Women's Association provided insights into the cultural aspects of living and working in Bali, as well as the instrumental role that members of the Bali Women's Association played at Sanglah Hospital in the aftermath of the bombing.

The local research assistants were paramount in the data collection process; as indicated earlier, they were the 'cultural interpreters' and were able to offer to the participants the choice to describe their experience in their preferred language (Bahasa Indonesian or Bahasa Balinese). This enabled the participants to feel as comfortable with the interview process as possible.

Two interview schedules were developed to be used in both Perth and Bali. The interview schedule consisted of two parts: the first related to demographic data; the second contained open-ended questions relating to key aspects of the participants' experiences and recollections regarding the Bali bombings of 2002. The interviews varied in length from 60 to 90 minutes.

The interview schedule was designed to elicit information based on the overarching aim of the study, which was to examine the multilayered effects and forms of support received by directly affected victims and their indirectly affected family members. Each in-depth interview took 1–1.5 hours. The second semi-structured interview schedule was developed for volunteer and professional responders. Both interview schedules included a section that collected basic demographic details, and the second section of the schedule was designed to encourage participants to talk openly around a set of guiding questions.

With such a sensitive subject matter, it was inevitable that some participants would become emotional during the interview process. A number of participants, both male and female, either became emotional and cried during the interview process or became very quiet. At this juncture the participants were offered some respite from the interview. However, only three requested the interview be suspended for a short time. Where there was participant discomfort during the interviews, time out was taken and participants were given the contact details of a person who would assist after the research process if they became unduly upset.

Following the interview the participants were thanked for their participation and an informal debriefing process occurred; this process was also extended at the end of each day to ensure the research assistants were not upset by the interviewing process. By using a translator and transcribers who were residents from the host country, the likelihood of 'gaining comparability of meanings' was greatly enhanced (Birbili, 2000, p. 3).

The study site of Perth, Western Australia

Perth, the capital city of Western Australia (Figure 2.3), is the most isolated capital city in the world and has a population of 1.6 million people (Australian Bureau of Statistics, 2009). As previously discussed, its Mediterranean climate allows for an outdoor lifestyle and a wide range of sporting activities, including Australian Rules Football. The study in Perth was centred on an amateur local club, some of whose members had engaged in what had become a local custom of travelling to Bali at the end of the playing season. It was during their trip to Bali in 2002 that the bombings took place.

Kingsley Amateur Football Club was formed in 1994, with a home ground at the Kingsley reserve in Perth, Western Australia. As its web site states, the club is built on 'good leadership with a family and community atmosphere' (Kingsley Amateur Football Club, 2010). The club has a local following, with many fund-raising activities taking place during the year to support the club, and most games are well attended. In 2002 the club had a successful year, reaching the season grand final.

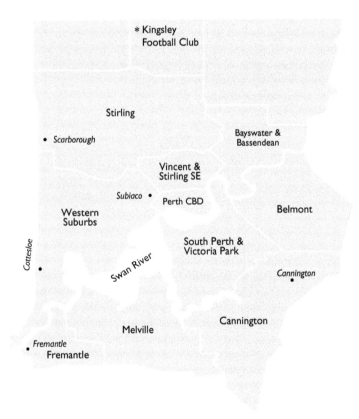

Figure 2.3 Map of Perth

Source: http://reiwa.com.au/AdvancedSearch/AdvancedSearchPage.aspx

The players had planned all year for their traditional end-of-season trip to Bali. In all 20 men went on the trip; 17 were players from the club, two were club officials and one was a friend of the players. Shortly after arriving the men had dinner and set off to visit the nightspots of Kuta. They commenced their evening in a discotheque and then went on to the popular Sari club. A few minutes after their arrival at the club, the bombing took place. Of the group, seven were killed in the bombing and 13 survived. The bombing had a devastating impact on the players and their families.

Recruitment of participants

In the Perth sample, 17 participants took part (Table 2.3).

The same criteria discussed previously were used with the Kingsley participants to exclude participants who may have been at psychological risk. Participants were again identified by using purposive, volunteer, opportunistic and snowball techniques. Two club committee members were enlisted to recruit the participants from Perth.

Collecting the data

Once again, contact was made with participants, an interview time was agreed upon and then the interviews were undertaken. All of the interviews were audio-taped, after seeking permission to do so. Specifics for each victim group are detailed as follows.

Primary-level victims (PLV) – Of the four males interviewed, three were players who had gone on the end-of-season football trip; the remaining interviewee was a friend of a football player who had joined the trip. Three of the interviews took place in the researcher's office and one in a participant's home.

Secondary-level victims (SLV) – All five of the participants were family members whose loved ones had been either killed or injured in the bombing. Two of the interviews took place in the participants' homes and three in the researcher's office. All participants lived in the inner suburbs of Perth.

Third-level victims (TLV) – Three of the volunteers interviewed were male volunteers who formed part of the support team from the Kingsley Football Club committee. One of the professionals interviewed was a male surgeon who had worked with many burns victims from Bali and Perth in the days following the

Table 2.3 Participants recruited for interviews – Kingsley

Primary Victims	Secondary Victims	Third-Level Volunteers	Third-Level Professionals	Key Informants
	3 Female			1 Female
4 Male	2 Male	3 Male	1 Male	3 Male

bombings, when victims were evacuated to Perth. Two of the interviews took place in the participants' offices, one in the participant's home and one in the researcher's office.

Key informants – Three key informants were interviewed. One was a government-employed departmental head, the second a professional media advisor and the third a local politician. Each of the key informants had acted as advisors to the Kingsley Football Club response committee. These interviews helped to gain further information regarding the decisions made by the committee, as well as the personal effect on the individuals concerned. One interview took place in the participant's office, and the remaining two in the participants' homes.

The same set of documents used for data collection in Bali were used in Kingsley; however, only the English version was applicable. Where there was participant discomfort during the interviews, time out was taken during the interview process and participants were given the contact details of a person who would assist after the research process if they became unduly upset. Following the interview, the participants were thanked for their participation.

Ethics

This study received ethics clearance from the administering institution. As the study was multi-site and involved both Indonesia and Australia it was important to abide by the appropriate guidelines; in this case they related to the Australian context, as the ethics clearance was gained from an Australian institution (Australian Government National Health and Medical Research Council, 2007). All participants provided informed consent, were told they could withdraw from the study at any time, that results would be shared and that they would be offered psychological help if needed.

Data analysis

Analysis of interviews was undertaken using framework analysis. There are five stages of data analysis in framework analysis, all of which were utilised to analyse the data in this study: familiarisation; identifying a thematic framework; indexing and charting; mapping; and interpretation (Dunican, 2005; Pope *et al*, 2000).

Familiarisation

Initially all the transcribed in-depth interviews were organised into first, second or third-level victim and country categories. The interview transcripts from Bali and Perth were read, organised and analysed separately. The aim was to gain familiarity with the participants, the information they shared and the initial emerging themes. At this stage consistent themes were listed in an informal way to assist with the process of interpretation of the data. A more formal method of thematic analysis was subsequently followed.

Identifying a thematic framework

In the next stage of the analysis, thematic framework analysis was used to organise and analyse the data. Each transcription was initially read line by line, as immersion in the raw data is an important first step in the framework approach to data analysis (Pope *et al*, 2000). The data was then coded to identify thematically related key ideas and themes. Initial coding helped to classify and assign meaning to the data without losing the context of the data (Pope *et al*, 2000). This was followed by focused coding to review and further refine the initial codes. Repeated ideas and themes emerged and the codes were reorganised and categorised into larger interconnecting themes (Silverman, 2006). The next stage required the themes and issues arising from the initial analysis of interviews to be examined for likenesses and differences with reference to the three core domains identified by the PWG framework (PWG, 2003) used to underpin the study and analysis. A framework grid was produced, with the three domains of human capacity, social capacity and culture and values on the vertical axis. The data was then categorised into major and minor themes and was listed on the horizontal axis (O'Connor, 2004).

Indexing and charting

This stage involved using an index systematically on all the data in textual form, by annotating the transcripts (Pope *et al*, 2000). The thematic framework was used as a basis for re-arrangement, and referencing the data within the three core domains of the PWG framework enabling listing and chart formation. The charts contained condensed summaries of the participants' views and experiences relating to the Bali bombings.

Mapping and interpretation

Finally, the charts were used to define concepts, plot the range of phenomena, create topologies and find associations between themes to provide meaning (Pope *et al*, 2000).

Quality criteria in the study

In studies using insightful and responsive techniques, the researcher must also be mindful that such techniques must also be scientifically rigorous. Rigour, or the trustworthiness of this study, was an important consideration from the outset. The criteria by which most qualitative research may be judged are credibility, confirmability and transferability (Houghton *et al*, 2013). Some consider trustworthiness to also be an important component, as it demonstrates important factors such as reliability and validity (Cohen and Crabtree, 2008). To enhance the credibility and overall trustworthiness of this study, a range of techniques was employed which included prolonged engagement, using participants' language, peer debriefing, participant checks, persistent observation and triangulation (Houghton *et al*, 2013).

Methodological triangulation

Methodological triangulation was utilised to improve the probability that the findings and interpretations would be considered credible and to augment the understanding of the study (Bekhet and Zauszniewski, 2012). Multiple data-gathering procedures were used, such as semi-structured interviews with three levels of victims and key informants, detailed observations, documentary data collection from newspapers and official reports and maintaining a reflective journal.

Use of an audit trail

An audit trail (Barusch *et al*, 2011) – an orderly and detailed description of the study – was produced for others to follow and replicate. The written field notes, daily reflective journals, personal notes, audio tapes of interviews and subsequent transcripts were well maintained to provide a comprehensive and open account of the research process in Bali and in Perth. The aim was to supply sufficient descriptive data to make similarity judgments possible and to facilitate transferability of the study (Brown, 2005) by providing 'thick' and detailed descriptions.

Member checking

The criterion for member checking was fulfilled by having a selection of transcripts assessed by independent transcribers to assess consistency and accuracy of interpretation. Respondent validation was also employed to enable cross-checking of emerging themes to determine accuracy (Silverman, 2006). A selection of trusted peers and the researcher's supervisor were consulted on numerous occasions throughout the research process for debriefing purposes and to validate the themes that evolved from the interview analysis.

The researcher presented the research methodology, findings and writings for peer group review and critique at professional meetings, conferences and colloquiums. As language should be used to transfer meaning (Vygotsky, cited in Poggenpoel and Myburg, 2005), to further enhance this process the language used within this study was deliberately devoid of technical jargon in an effort to promote understanding and validation by the reader.

Use of a reflective journal

Cohen and Crabtree (2008, p. 333) suggest that one of the 'hallmarks' of good research is reflexive processing through the use of reflective journal keeping on the part of the researcher. The use of a reflective journal is considered an essential component of any research study. Reflective journals ensure we talk about our own 'thoughts, beliefs and behaviours' (Janesick, 1999, p. 521). By maintaining detailed notes during the interview process, rich information and observations were recorded about the participants, the interview process and the researcher's impressions. By writing 'in the moment', information was fresh and original (Silverman, 2006). The journal also provided information that continued to help with cultural understanding. Each evening, as part of a 'letting go of the day's routine', a second journal was written, cataloguing situations, positive and negative events and interactions, more general observations, the daily course of progressive decision-making and reflections on the interview process. This journal became part of an essential nightly routine and debriefing process for the researcher. These reflections, notes, observations and cathartic revelations were later matched with data elicited from the interviews to identify key factors.

Summary

A detailed description of the research methodology has been described. An audit trail has been provided containing full details of the research approach, conceptual framework, research design, data collection methods and analysis techniques employed to ensure validity, reliability and ethical consideration. The primary objective was to enhance the credibility and overall transparency of this study and to confirm the qualitative approach as an appropriate paradigm for this study.

Chapter 3 will present analysis of the socio-demographic data of both the Balinese and Perth-based participants.

References

Australian Bureau of Statistics (2009). *Australian social trends, March 2009*. Retrieved 20 Aug 2014 from http://www.abs.gov.au/ausstats/abs

Australian Government, National Health and Medical Research Council (NHMRC) (2007). *Australian code for the responsible conduct of research. R 39*. Retrieved 20 Aug 2014 from http://www.nhmrc.gov.au/publications/synopses/r39syn.htm

Barusch, A., Gringeri, C., and George, M. (2011). Rigor in qualitative social work research: A review of strategies used in published articles. *Social Work Research, 35*(1), 11–19. Retrieved 20 Aug 2014 from http://search.proquest.com/docview/858669781?accountid=10382

Bekhet, K., and Zauszniewski, J. (2012). Methodological triangulation: An approach to understanding data. *Nurse Researcher, 20*(2), 40–43. Retrieved 20 Aug 2014 from http://search.proquest.com/docview/1325690432?accountid=10382

Birbili, M. (2000). Translating from one language to another. *Social Research Update 31*, 1–7. Retrieved 20 Aug 2014 from http://sru.surrey.ac.uk

Brown, J. D. (2005). Characteristics of sound qualitative research. *Journal of Testing and Evaluation SIG Newsletter, 9*(2), 31–33. Retrieved 20 Aug 2014 from http://jalt.org/test/bro_22.htm

Capaldi, E. J., and Proctor, R. W. (2005). Is the world of qualitative inquiry a proper guide for psychological research? *American Journal of Psychology, 118*(2), 251–269.

Cohen, D. J., and Crabtree, B. F. (2008). Evaluative criteria for qualitative research in health care: Controversies and recommendations. *Annals of Family Medicine, 6*(4), 331–339.

Creswell, J. W. (2007). *Qualitative inquiry and research design: Choosing from five traditions* (2nd ed.). Thousand Oaks, CA: Sage.

Daly, J., Willis, K., Small, R., Green, J., Welch, N., Kealy, M., and Hughes, E. (2007). A hierarchy of evidence for assessing qualitative health research. *Journal of Clinical Epidemiology, 60*, 43–49.

Dunican, E. (2005, June). A framework for evaluating qualitative research methods in computer programming education. In P. Romero, J. Good, E. Acosta Chaparro and S. Bryant (Eds), *Proceedings of the 17th Workshop of the Psychology of Programming Interest Group*. Sussex: Sussex University, 225–257. Retrieved 20 Aug 2014 from http://www.ppig.org/papers/17th-dunican.pdf

Houghton, C., Casey, D., Shaw, D., and Murphy, K. (2013). Rigour in qualitative case-study research. *Nurse Researcher, 20*(4), 12–17. Retrieved 20 Aug 2014 from http://search.proquest.com/docview/1317920491?accountid=10382

Inter-Agency Standing Committee (IASC) 4th Working Draft (2006). *Guidance on mental health and psychosocial support in emergency settings*. Inter-Agency Standing Committee, 4–80. Retrieved 20 Aug 2014 from http://www.who.int/mental_health/emergencies/guidelinesiasc_mental_health_psychosocial_june_2007.pdf

Janesick, V. J. (1999). A journal about journal writing as a qualitative research technique: History, issues, and reflections. *Qualitative Inquiry, 5*, 505–524.

Kingsley Amateur Football Club (2010). Retrieved 20 Aug 2014 from kingsleyamateur footballclub.com.au/index.php

Lloyd-Jones, M. (2004). Application of systematic review methods to qualitative research practical issues. *Journal of Advanced Nursing, 48*(3), 271–278.

Longden, B. (2001). *Leaving college early – a qualitative case study*. (Report on research project for Higher Education Funding Council for England). 1–68. Retrieved 20 Aug 2014 from http://www.ulster.ac.uk/star/resources/hefce_report.pdf

Malik, R. (2012). Ancient outpost of Hinduism thrives in modern times. Retrieved 20 Aug 2014 from http://www.hinduismtoday.com/modules/smartsection/item.php?itemid=5267

Noor, K. B. M. (2008). Case study: A strategic research methodology. *American Journal of Applied Science, 5*(11), 1602–1604.

O'Connor, P. (2004). The conditionality of status: Experience-based reflections on the insider/outsider issue. *Australian Geographer, 35*(2), 169–176.

Pitchforth, E., and Van Teijlingen, E. (2005). International public health research involving interpreters: a case study from Bangladesh. *BMC Public Health, 5*(1), 71–78. Retrieved 20 Aug 2014 from http://www.biomedcentral.com/1471-2458/5/71/

Poggenpoel, M., and Myburgh, C. P. (2005). Obstacles in qualitative research: Possible solutions. *Education, 126*(2), 304–311.

Pope, C., Ziebland, S., and Mays, N. (2000). Qualitative research in health care: Analysing qualitative data. *British Medical Journal, 320*(7227), 114–116.

Psychosocial Working Group (PWG) (2003). *Psychosocial intervention in complex emergencies: A framework for practice*. Working Paper. Centre for International Health Studies, Queen Margaret University, Edinburgh.

Silverman, D. (2006). *Interpreting qualitative data: Methods for analyzing talk, text, and interaction*. London: Sage Publications Ltd.

Strang, A. B., and Ager, A. (2001). *Building a conceptual framework for psychosocial intervention in complex emergencies: reporting on the work of the Psychosocial Working Group*, 1–6. Centre for International Health Studies, Queen Margaret University, Edinburgh.

Tellis, W. (1997). Application of a case study methodology. *The Qualitative Report, 3*(3), 1–18.

Yin, R. K. (2003). *Applications of case study research* (3rd ed.). Newbury Park, CA: Sage.

YKIDS/Yayasan Kuta International Disaster Scholarship (2002). Retrieved 20 Aug 2014 from http://www.alfoundation.org/charity/alfinbali/YKIP-YKIDS-Trust-Fund_16

YKIP (2007). *YKIP's journey: The first five years*. Bali, Indonesia: Annika Linden Foundation and Reset.

Chapter 3

The effects on victims in Bali

Introduction

In this chapter the data from the primary and secondary victims in Bali are presented. The information is categorised under the following themes: the effects of terrorist attacks; primary and secondary-level victims of terrorist attacks; post-traumatic stress among victims; effects on primary, secondary and third-level victims; community-level effects; interventions using a psychosocial approach to support vulnerable groups; resilience; and post-traumatic growth.

The effects

As discussed, the effects of terrorist attacks and disasters are multi-layered and not limited to the physical or psychological. It is not uncommon for individual victims to report effects such as insomnia, nightmares, suppressed emotions, the use of drugs and alcohol and feelings of anger (Meisenhelder and Marcum, 2009). While most of the effects reported are now viewed as 'normal reactions' to a very abnormal situation (Fetter, 2005; Forbes *et al*, 2009), the effects are distressing and unpleasant, with some victims reporting significant distress some years after the event. Nightmares, for example, are not an unusual response to trauma, as they often contain information related to the traumatic experience. Nightmares alone are difficult for the victim to experience; however, they can also lead to a spill-over effect in which sleep disturbances and an increase in depression and anxiety-related symptoms are reported, which compound the victim's problems (Davis *et al*, 2007). Symptoms such as difficulty sleeping and unpleasant memories of the event can, however, be termed 'transient' symptoms, from which most people recover over time (Bonanno *et al*, 2007; Yehudi and Hyman, 2005).

Increased alcohol and drug use and smoking following a terrorist attack have been well documented; for example, following the 9/11 attacks people were found to be self-medicating as a way of relaxing or being able to cope (DiMaggio *et al*, 2009; Moore *et al*, 2004; Vlahov *et al*, 2006). It is also not unusual for victims caught up in traumatic events to exhibit strong feelings of anger, particularly towards the perpetrators of the attack (Orth *et al*, 2008). In a study of coping and emotional reactions in the aftermath of 9/11, anger was the predominant emotion expressed by the recipients (Orth *et al*, 2008). Although some studies consider high levels of anger to be symptomatic of post-traumatic stress disorder (PTSD) (Orth *et al*, 2008), others positively correlate it with emotional growth and positive coping, and view it as a necessary outlet for victims' distress. In other words, in this way victims have a positive and 'active engagement with a stressor' (Park *et al*, 2008, p. 307).

Since 9/11 the effects of terrorist attacks have been a primary focus of interest in the literature. Prior to this, studies on the effects of manmade or natural disasters concentrated mainly on the psychological distress experienced by victims (Adams and Boscarino, 2005; Neria *et al*, 2008). The most popular focus in past research has been PTSD, with more than 30,000 citations listed in the US National Center for PTSD database in 2006 (National Center for PTSD, 2009). However, this is just one of the many types or 'layers' of effects with which individuals may present following a disaster. Following the Bali bombings, the multilayered effects reported by first-level victims included feelings of anger, depression and anxiety, but also elements of post-traumatic growth (PTG), such as feeling closer to their families and revaluating what was important to them (Brookes, 2010).

Primary and secondary-level victims of terrorist attacks

When disasters such as the Boston bombing (2011), the London bombing (2005) and the Bali bombings of 2002 and 2005 occur, it is to be expected that those directly at the scene will be affected and traumatised; however, it is now recognised that there are other victims who also get caught up in the terror of the event. A review of the literature suggests there are between four and six identified levels of victims (Buesnel, 2004; Taylor, 1990), although the majority of the studies refer to three levels of victims: primary, secondary and third-level (Alexander, 2005; Rao, 2006). The victims are usually classified with regard to their proximity to the disaster: primary-level victims are identified as those who have been killed or injured, and are therefore directly involved by being in or around the vicinity of the attack; secondary-level victims are defined as family and friends of primary-level victims; and third-level victims are the volunteer or professional responders who usually assist the first two levels of victims in the aftermath of the attack.

There are variations on this approach, with the primary-level victim classification now including those who have suffered property damage and the secondary-level classification including professional responders such as fire and ambulance personnel and volunteers. The third-level victim classification may now include tertiary or vicarious victims of terrorism, such as ordinary citizens not directly caught up in the act, but who have experienced fear as a result of it (Cohen, 2002), often as a result of seeing the carnage on television or reading about it in the newspapers.

Other categories of victims in the community who are indirect victims of the attacks have also been identified. This includes office workers and people who live in the area close to the attack. A significant study by Osinubi *et al* (2008) following the 9/11 attacks highlighted the traumatising effects on office workers who were not directly involved, in that they neither witnessed the event nor were in the vicinity at the time of the impacts. Two years after the event, the 369 workers were assessed using a 170-item Likert-scale questionnaire. An unexpected finding was reports of high rates of 'new onset psychological difficulties' such as 'depression, anxiety disorders and panic attacks' (Osinubi *et al*, 2008, p. 113). It is thought this occurred in part because the office workers were less likely to have access to the psychological or counselling programmes that are usually available to directly affected victims (Osinubi *et al*, 2008).

There has been an increase, albeit small, in research which focuses on the effects on volunteers who respond to the call for help in a complex disaster. This has resulted in growing awareness that being involved in a disaster response as a volunteer or a professional responder can have detrimental effects. A number of studies exploring this topic took place following Hurricane Katrina in 2005[1] (Adams, 2007; Swygard and Stafford, 2009) and after 9/11 (Kinsel and Thomasgard, 2008). There was no shortage of participants to study following 9/11: it has been calculated that 30,000 volunteers responded to calls for help (Brand *et al*, 2008). An increase in PTSD symptoms has been linked with first-time responders, who were unlikely to have been previously exposed to the sights and sounds of a disaster-type situation (Park *et al*, 2008).

In the same study there was a suggestion of a protective effect if volunteers had previous exposure to emergency situations and disaster training (Park *et al*, 2008), although it wasn't clear how much training or how much exposure was required to produce this effect. However, it appeared the risk of PTSD was reduced if some control was exerted to reduce the amount of time first-time responders spent in the disaster situation. Adams (2007) challenges this finding in a study which explored the negative effects reported in the aftermath of a disaster situation by trained volunteer responders attached to the Red Cross and other smaller organisations. Members of the Red Cross received training as an important component of their membership and would, if the previously cited study is correct, be expected to have a reduced incidence of PTSD symptoms. However, the study found that the training received by the responders did not have a significant protective effect.

Apart from spending too much time at a disaster site, factors such as living near a disaster site (as many did in 9/11) and indirect exposure as a result of working to support victims and their family members during long shifts are said to contribute to first responders' distress (McCaslin *et al*, 2005). The effects in the 9/11 responders were compounded by the fact that a significant number were subjected to additional levels of distress as they lived and worked in the area which had been targeted. It is therefore not surprising that they reported high levels of psychological distress (McCaslin *et al*, 2005). As so many people can be identified as victims of attacks, the view is confirmed that terrorists aim to go beyond the immediate and, as Jenkins (as cited in Howe, 2006, p. 1) suggests, 'to want a lot of people watching, not a lot of people dead'. In other words, the aim is to promote a high level of fear among members of the general population not directly injured in the terrorist event.

Conversely, there are other studies that report on the beneficial effects of working in a disaster area. For example, a longitudinal qualitative study of 9/11 volunteers by Steffen and Fothergill (2009) surveyed participants over two data collection periods and found that benefits included 'personal healing, improvements to the volunteers' self-concept, and increased engagement in the community in non-disaster times' (p. 29). The benefits were not limited to the time of the attack but were reported some three years after 9/11. Although there is a growing body of research regarding the adverse effects experienced by volunteer responders, it is not extensive. It is likely that those with certain personalities will benefit from their volunteering experiences, some may be adversely affected and others may report a combination of both. This is an area worthy of further attention by researchers.

Post-traumatic stress disorder among victims

Previous research investigating terrorist attacks has focused on the individual and has shown that many victims experience some form of reaction to the attack. This can range from slight to moderate distress through to symptoms of post-traumatic stress (Mansdorf, 2008), which was first categorised in the Diagnostic and Statistical Manual of Mental Health Disorders in 1980. Following the attacks of 9/11, there was an increase in the number of studies that examined the psychological symptoms of post-traumatic stress in victims, particularly in the immediate aftermath of a disaster (Boscarino and Adams, 2007; Jayasinghe *et al*, 2008; Tuchner *et al*, 2010). The result of the studies was that clinicians recommended early psychological interventions for almost all persons exposed to a traumatic event.

PTSD occurs when victims have been exposed to an extreme event such as a terrorist attack and is characterised by a number of symptoms, including fear, helplessness and horror. The diagnosis is usually confirmed when it is accompanied by symptoms and signs of hyper-arousal such as anger, difficulty falling asleep and difficulty concentrating, which last for longer than a month. Additionally, the person may revisit the event by way of recurrent distressful images, thoughts or perceptions (Agronick *et al*, 2007; National Center for PTSD, 2009). There is a growing interest in the literature in the correlation of initial peri-traumatic reactions such as fear, helplessness and horror with the eventual development of PTSD symptomology (Lawyer *et al*, 2006).

Interestingly, a key study surrounding the London suicide bombings, known as 7/7, in July 2005 found survivors' accounts fell into two time periods accompanied by two different sets of symptoms: namely those symptoms that occurred on the day of the bombing, such as shock and horror, and post-7/7 PTSD-type symptoms which were accompanied by feelings of disconnection from others, particularly those who had not been involved in the bombing (Wilson *et al*, 2012, p. 8). Research is continuing in this area, as it is hoped it will lead to additional information which may enable public information campaigns to target those most at risk following an attack and help formulate more effective post-attack interventions. The concept of post-traumatic stress disorder is a topic which has dominated past literature and has been a focus of controversy, with even experts in the disaster response field failing to reach consensus on the subject (Van Ommeron *et al*, 2005).

In research which does recognise the disorder, it has been suggested that individuals may be more resilient than was perhaps previously thought. Following 9/11, one group of residents in New York initially exhibited moderate distress and only a few PTSD symptoms, which improved quite quickly to mild distress, until eventually they were demonstrating no distress or PTSD symptoms at all (Norris *et al*, 2009). This indicates that initial symptoms may reduce in some individuals, given time. PTSD and its effects in victims are explained further in the following sections.

Effects on primary-level victims

In the aftermath of the 2002 Bali bombings, 9/11 and the 2004 tsunami in the Indian Ocean, numerous victims required immediate and ongoing support. The effects of such an event at the individual and community levels are complex and often multi-layered, and have already been discussed. The main current focus of research in this area is the psychological effects on the victims, as they are unexpectedly disconnected from their normal routine and their 'beliefs about themselves and their world [are] forever altered' (Miller, 2004, p. 2). Following the 9/11 attacks and the Indian Ocean tsunami, the disasters' psychological impacts on directly affected primary-level victims were examined (DiMaggio *et al*, 2009; Mitka, 2008) with a particular focus on PTSD and its psychological sequelae, which highlighted reported symptoms such as nightmares, sleep disturbance, flashbacks and dissociation (Giosan *et al*, 2009; Pfeffer *et al*, 2009).

Effects on secondary-level victims

Increasingly, research is being conducted into effects on secondary-level victims. Secondary-level victims can include family members and friends who gave support to primary-level family members and those who were adversely affected by witnessing the attack on television. Family members of primary-level victims receive second-hand exposure to the events by virtue of having to hear repeated recollections of the events of the attack (Gregerson, 2007; Pulido, 2007; Shalev *et al*, 2006). Family friends and community members rallied to help the victims in all of the 'ground zeros'. They too were affected by the events and became secondary-level victims.

This indirect exposure can result in the same effects previously discussed as occurring in first-level victims, namely reoccurring painful memories, difficulty in falling or staying asleep, fear and nightmares. Victims may also describe shock, numbness and disbelief, all symptoms that have been listed in previous studies as symptoms of PTSD (Bride, 2007; Muñoz et al, 2004; Rao, 2006; Watchorn, 2001). Other studies consider suppression of emotions a useful coping mechanism which is necessary to promote emotional equilibrium at the time (Rosenthal, cited in Holmes, 2005, p. 434) and allows the victims to cope with the many roles they have to take up.

Painful reoccurring memories, known as 'flashbulb memories', of the event are not an unusual consequence for secondary-level victims (Perina, 2002, p. 1). They too are caught up in the events by having a close family member involved and they are often required to play an intense supportive role with that person, despite their own high levels of distress. Some researchers are of the opinion that after a year the memories of the event will alter, as the emotional reactions to the event are remembered less well than the 'where I was when I found out'-type non-emotional memories (Hirst et al, 2009, p. 163).

The findings that emerged from the study of the Bali bombings are presented in the following three chapters. This chapter presents the effects on the primary (PLV) and secondary-level victims (SLV) from Bali. First, a socio-demographic profile of the participants is presented and described; second, presentation of the data from the semi-structured interviews gives voice to the personal experiences of primary and secondary-level victims.

Socio-demographic profiles of the participants in Bali

Age and gender

All study participants were adults over the age of 18 years who had either been injured in the bombing, namely primary-level victims, or were family members or friends of those who had been killed or injured, namely secondary-level victims. In total, PLVs numbered ten, of whom five (50 per cent) were female and five were male; SLVs numbered 11, of whom all (100 per cent) were female. The majority of both PLVs and SLVs were in the age range 37–42 years (Table 3.3).

Marital status

The majority of participants interviewed in both the PLV and SLV groups were married, or had been married. Of the ten PLVs, nine (90 per cent) were married and one (10 per cent) was separated; of the 11 SLVs, five were widowed (46 per cent) and six (54 per cent) were married.

Widows

Of the SLV participants, five were widowed. Clearly, the loss of a male partner was extremely distressful for the women. In Bali the loss of a husband and main bread-winner is associated with a myriad of extra pressures for the women. One widow interviewed for this study stated she did not venture out on her own at night to community events for almost two years after the loss of her husband, as she thought other women might think she wanted to steal their husbands (Widow 3, personal communication, 22 February 2008). Delayed marriage, divorce, single parenting and the title of widow are not well accepted in Indonesian society due to entrenched social stigma (Jones and Gubhaju, 2008). For the widows, this altered status and the responsibility of becoming a single parent added to their considerable distress. As they took on the role of primary carer in the family, they had to urgently find a source of regular income and financial support. With the global economic down-turn and its impact on tourism, it was difficult for the women to find gainful work yet eventually all of the women found employment, with the majority working at a local co-operative; one widow subsequently left to return to work as a teacher.

Number of children

All of the children (PLV, n = 17; SLV, n = 11) came from families in which the parents were married, reflecting the cultural trend, as having children out of marriage is very rare in Balinese society (Hirschman and Teerawichitchainan, 2003). The larg-est number of children in a single family was eight, with the majority of families having three children or fewer. This correlates with the total fertility rate (TFR) of 2.21 recorded in the 2007 Bali survey by Sekilas Bali (Badan Pusat Statistik, 2009). The Balinese TFR is lower than the national Indonesian average of 3.8.

Employment

In the period prior to the bombing, six (60 per cent) of the ten PLV participants were employed. As they were injured mainly as a result of being employed in and around the Sari club and Paddy's bar, it would follow that this would be reflected in a high figure of employment. The 11 SLVs were all female, with seven (64 per cent) reporting that they had been employed prior to the bombing. Post-bombing, two of the PLV participants in Bali no longer worked for the same employer as had been the case prior to the bombing, but five continued working with their previous employers. Overall only two SLV participants still worked for the same employer; nine were not with the same employer or were unemployed.

Income characteristics

Of the PLV, seven households disclosed a regular income and three declined to comment. Two victims were earning an excellent wage by Balinese standards: one, a businessman, was earning A$1,400 per month, and another approximately

A$900 per month. Of the rest, five were earning below A$400 per month. In the SLV group, ten households disclosed an income and one declined to comment. Two were self-employed and running well-established businesses; however, the majority of the women in this group (n = 5) were earning less than A$400 and three had no fixed income and relied on family support. The majority of participants in both groups were earning less than A$400 a month.

Religion

In the SLV participant group the predominant religion was Hindu (64 per cent, n = 7); the remaining participants (36 per cent, n = 4) were Muslim prior to the bombing. The majority of Bali's population is Hindu (Edelhäuser, 2005). Hinduism has a long history in Bali, having arrived via Java and India between the eighth and sixteenth centuries (Bali 123, n.d.). The mainly Hindu population has found a duality of purpose in their religion: it not only serves a spiritual need, particularly in a time of crisis, but also gives them a collective identity, status and a political platform to enable them to be heard without harsh military interventions or oppression (Howe, 2001).

In comparison to the SLV group, only 30 per cent (n = 3) of PLV participants followed the Hindu religion, with the majority, 50 per cent (n = 5), being Muslim and 20 per cent (n = 2) Christian. In general, the Muslim community in Bali is in the minority; however, a high proportion of rural Muslims, known as 'Bali Siam' or 'Bali Muslims', are descendants of long-standing island populations (Pedersen, 2009). Recently the number of immigrant and 'new' Muslims in Bali has been growing steadily, with a report in 2000 indicating the population of Muslims had grown by 6 per cent in the preceding decade (Pedersen, 2009). During the SLV interviews, two previously Hindu and Muslim participants indicated that they had changed their religion to Christianity, reportedly as a result of their near-death experience and the support they received from Christian groups at the time of the bombings.

Level of education

The demographic data also examined the highest level of education attained by the participants. Of the PLV group, two (10 per cent) had received primary-level education only, six (60 per cent) had received secondary-level education and one (10 per cent) had attended tertiary-level education. Of the SLV, three (27 per cent) had received primary-level education only, six (54 per cent) had received secondary education and two had received tertiary education. Of the two SLV participants who had received tertiary education, both came from middle-income families and were now involved in professional occupations and receiving relatively high incomes compared to the rest of the population. In both groups the majority of participants had received secondary-level education, probably because of the great emphasis on education in Bali, with many

Table 3.1 Demographic characteristics of primary-level victims – Bali

Demographic and descriptive variables	Total Participants n = 10
Age	
31–36 years	4
37–42 years	5
43–48 years	1
Gender	
Female	5
Male	5
Marital Status	
Separated	1
Married	9
Religion	
Hindu	3
Muslim	5
Christian	2
Education	
Primary	2
Secondary	6
Tertiary	1
Employment	
Employed	7
Unemployed	3
Income	
AUD $ 200 to AUD $ 400	5
AUD $ 400 to AUD $ 900	1
AUD $ 900 to AUD $ 1400	1
Did not respond	3

parents viewing education as a way to escape poverty (participant discussions, 2008). See Tables 3.1 and 3.2 for details.

Forms of support

The ten PLVs and 11 SLVs received medical, counselling, community and spiritual support from a number of sources and in varying amounts (see Table 3.3). Of the PLV group, five (50 per cent) participants received medical support, mainly for burns and eye injuries, and five (50 per cent) received counselling support. Two (20 per cent) received religious support and one (10 per cent) received community support. Of the SLV participants, eight (62 per cent) received counselling support and eight (62 per cent) received religious support; seven (54 per cent) received medical support, and six (46 per cent) received community support.

Counselling and religious support were found to be the forms of support most utilised by the Bali participants. Medical support had also been widely used by both groups. A number of the PLV participants described receiving care initially

Table 3.2 Demographic characteristics of secondary-level victims – Bali

Demographic and descriptive variables	Total Participants n = 11
Age	
31–36 years	2
37–42 years	5
43–48 years	2
49–54 years	1
55–60 years	1
Gender	
Female	11
Male	0
Marital Status	
Married	6
Widowed	5
Religion	
Hindu	7
Muslim	4
Education	
Primary	3
Secondary	6
Tertiary	2
Employment	
Employed	7
Unemployed	4
Monthly Income	
A$200–400	5
A$7,000–9,000	1
A$9,000–10,000	1
Did not respond	1
Varied family support	3

at Sanglah hospital for their burns and blast injuries. The most severely injured were transferred to Australia for treatment in Perth hospitals. A number of the severely injured also received support in the initial aftermath from their community and, eventually, local NGOs. Often this support was in the form of food, or small amounts of money to buy food, as this group of people were unable to work due to their psychological and physical injuries. The SLV group reported similar support, as they had little or no money in the form of savings or government support with which to buy basic food staples. The community also supplied support for funeral rituals and ceremonies, which form an important part of the traditional way of life in the villages of Bali.

In both groups a number of participants (61 per cent of PLVs and 50 per cent of SLVs, see Table 3.3) took up the counselling support offered. The counselling was delivered in the main by psychiatrists at the hospital in Bali, while in Perth it was mainly in the form of psychologists provided by the government, Red Cross

Table 3.3 Forms of support received by participant victims – Bali

	Medical	Counselling	Community	Spiritual
PLVs	5	5	1	2
SLVs	7	8	6	8

and volunteers. The Bali participants indicated the psychiatrists' fees were paid by a number of the NGOs set up for support purposes post-bombing.

Summary

In Bali, analysis revealed the participants had additional stressors attributed to the effects of the bombing, apart from the loss or injury of a loved one or injury to themselves. Due to the downturn in tourism, the economic costs of the bombing for Bali and for the participants were extensive: as a result of it, many lost their jobs and were living below the poverty line. For the widows in the SLV group there were additional hardships as they had to deal with their altered status in Balinese society, the responsibilities of single parenthood and the need to earn a living within an economically distressed community. The predominant religion of the participants was Hindu (64 per cent), and with this came spiritual support during the time of the crisis and a collective identity with their Hindu neighbours, friends and family.

Analysis of interview data: Bali

The following section presents analysis of the data from the semi-structured interviews conducted. Strang and Ager (2003), two key members of the PWG, extended its conceptual framework and enhanced our understanding of what constitutes psychosocial well-being, with reference to appropriate interventions and the importance of community engagement. They suggest that a commonality in any form of disaster is that it 'diminishes or disrupts' a community's resources and that, in response, the community will strengthen and utilise the resources it has (Strang and Ager, 2003, p. 3).

Drawing on Strang and Ager's (2003) extension of the psychosocial framework, the term *disrupted resources* was used to describe factors that had a negative impact on the participants' lives, families, friends and the wider community they lived in. The term *reinforced resources* was used to map the many resources within the victims' family, friendship circles and community networks which were utilised to provide support. The resources are highlighted within the three domains of human capacity, social ecology and culture and values. The effectiveness with which resources are utilised by victims is an indicator of the extent of their resilience (PWG, 2003). It is suggested that following terrorist attacks, linkages within the three domains are activated

(PWG, 2003), and this is discussed in the context of primary and secondary-level participants in this study. Further, the multi-layered effects and support experienced by the victims are discussed.

This section commences with an examination of the domain of human capacity, also termed human capital. Strang and Ager (2003, p. 3) have defined human capacity as 'the physical and mental health of community members, their existing skills and knowledge, and their household livelihoods', and argue that complex emergency situations can lead to a reduction in human capacity at the individual and community levels. For example, as a consequence of an individual's injuries, the community is deprived of an individual's personal resources and skills due to the need for that person to withdraw, either temporarily or permanently, from community life so as to recover physically and psychologically (Strang and Ager, 2003).

Human capacity

The human capacity domain was used to examine and organise the Bali participants' descriptions of the effects of the bombing and the types of support they received. Within the sphere of disrupted resources, two main themes (effects and reactions) and three sub-themes (psychological, economic distress and fear) emerged from the analysis of the interviews, while two main themes (reflections and suggestions) and four sub-themes (communicating with friends and neighbours, practical and economic support, counselling and employment, no more bombs) were revealed within the reinforced resources context. These findings are illustrated diagrammatically in Figure 3.1.

Disrupted resource I: effects

Sub-theme: psychological effect

The psychological effect of the bombing on the primary-level victims was extensive. As a primary aim of a terrorist attack is to inculcate fear at the individual and community levels (Saul, 2008) it is not surprising that in the aftermath of the attack the Balinese victims described symptoms of depression, suicidal ideation and loss of self-confidence. As most lived near the disaster zone and had received injuries due to the attack, the stress they experienced in the aftermath was at a macro level (Richman *et al*, 2008, p. 114). A participant vividly described the rush of emotions she felt following the bombing, which she described as lasting for six months after the event. In most cases, if symptoms last for longer than a month, the person is more likely to be assessed and diagnosed with PTSD (Vijay-kumar *et al*, 2006).

Feeling sad and absent-minded and withdrawing from society were important indicators that this participant required further professional help, which she did eventually receive:

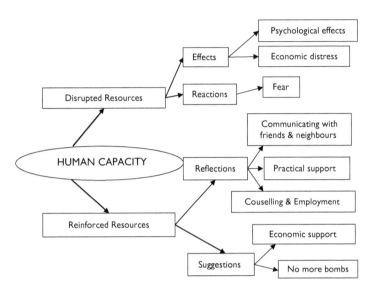

Figure 3.1 Human capacity – Bali

I [was] feeling helpless, I can't believe it, a bad dream, angry, sad, absent minded. It lasted for six months . . . I isolate[d] myself. After that I receive[d] therapy.

(Female victim)

The following participant described how he became withdrawn and depressed, partially due to his extensive burns and hearing loss. He also believed his friends had rejected him when he most needed them. His apparent withdrawal from society and the isolating effects of his deafness would have reduced this partici-pant's overall quality of life, and he lost confidence in his abilities. Most survivors will 'feel lonely, isolated and afraid' (Rao, 2006, p. 505), and need the comfort, support and reassurance of others (MacGeorge *et al*, 2004; Vijaykumar *et al*, 2006; Walsh, 2007).

I feel so shy and lose self-confidence. I feel my friends reject me.

(Injured male)

Another victim felt that life wasn't worth living and wanted to commit suicide. Fortunately this feeling subsided with the support of his family and friends. For him, the comfort and support of others was a crucial part of his recovery process:

Two months after the bomb blast I wanted to commit suicide. . . Talking to family and friends help[ed].

(Injured male)

Sub-theme: economic distress

In the weeks following the bombing, the occupancy rate of hotels in Bali fell; the impact on the Indonesian economy was estimated to be in the region of 0.5–2 per cent of GDP in the period 2002–2003 (Asian Development Bank, 2003, p. 4). As a result, many hotels and restaurants closed for business and laid off staff. The average weekly wage for hotel workers in Bali is A$36 and no unemployment or welfare benefits are provided by the government. While hospital fees and medicines were covered by the government, on leaving hospital the victims and their families had little or no income. There were times when they did not have sufficient rice or other food to feed their family, or money to purchase petrol for their motorbikes to enable them to attend job interviews. This meant they were dependent on NGOs, family members and friends for food and monetary donations. For the victims, the economic effect compounded their physical and psychological injuries. The following accounts highlight the victims' experiences under the theme of disrupted economic resources.

> I lose the job. It affects my daily life a bit hard because I don't have steady job.
>
> (Injured male)

This victim's account documents how many were unable to afford daily basic food and were worried about their survival and where they would find a job. They returned to their villages as they knew the community would rally round to help them. This was an excellent example of how a village would 'draw on its own resources' to 'meet their own needs' (PWG, 2003, p. 2):

> The most [effect] about economic aspect was so bad. Because the source [of jobs] was the tourists. Everyone complain about the economic problem. My neighbours concern re economic aspects, whether they could survive. If not working in Bali where can I get job? Many neighbours [went] back to their village as [they] could not afford daily life anymore.
>
> (Injured male)

Disrupted resource 2: reactions

Sub-theme: fear

Three of the participants reported being fearful in certain situations, such as when hearing loud sounds or during thunderstorms, which, given their experiences, would not be unusual. In this instance the terrorists had certainly instilled ongoing fear and anxiety in the victims. A female participant referred to the severe weather that Bali experiences in the wet season and described how she still gets frightened during thunderstorms. Her ongoing fears also result in her avoiding attending large gatherings for special ceremonies, such as prior to *Nyepi* day.

Instead she leaves Bali and attends the ceremonies in her hometown of Jakarta, where she feels she and her children will be safe. The second quote below is from a participant who is also afraid of ceremonial occasions in Bali, as firecrackers are often a part of the celebrations and they remind him of the sound of the bombs going off at ground zero.

> Now [in 2008] sometimes if there is thunder I feel afraid if it [is] like a bomb. Now I [am] just thinking about my children. If there is a special ceremony I prefer to go to my home in Jakarta.
>
> (Injured female)

> I am still afraid [in 2008] at Imlek [Chinese New Year] or other ceremonies because of terrorist[s].
>
> (Injured male)

Reinforced resource I: reflections

Sub-theme: talking to friends and neighbours

As discussed, most of the victims in Bali had overwhelming financial difficulties due to loss of earnings and the downturn in tourism. Participants described the types of support they received in the aftermath of the crisis. In many cases the support of friends and neighbours was recognised as extremely beneficial. This included emotional support in the form of a chat about their problems, especially when the victims were feeling sad and lonely. Friends and neighbours also supplied crucial help with childcare when the participants needed to look for work. This type of positive social support is now seen as a crucial element in an individual's recovery.

When victims are able to access and share their experiences with others, a sense of communal openness evolves which can help mediate the effects of a disaster (Steury et al, 2004) and decrease their levels of depression, and which has been correlated with an increase in levels of resilience (Moscardino et al, 2010). If victims experience a low level of social support following an attack, an increase in depressive symptomology has been observed (Moscardino et al, 2010). The following statements are examples of how friends and neighbours rallied to emotionally support the participants.

> When I meet my sister I usually talk about life, talked about my children who often get sick. My sister sometimes gives me food [and] money and look[s] after my children.
>
> (Wife of injured male)

> I feel better after I talk with my best friend.
>
> (Injured female)

I feel my neighbours' moral support [is] really useful to me because I look after the two of my children by myself.

(Injured female)

The most useful support was moral support from my neighbours.

(Injured male)

Friends often come, they pick me up and [we] went to [a] friend's house or camping with many friends.

(Injured male)

Sub-theme: practical support

For some participants practical support in the form of food, money and help during special ceremonies was very important, as they had little money and what they did have was required to feed the family. Help was particularly important at ceremony times as in Bali these are elaborate and expensive affairs, which all members of the village usually attend.

I receive help with white material, rice and money and they putting energy [volunteer] into ceremonies.

(Mother-in-law of victim)

My neighbours at the village came to ceremony. Neighbours gave money and rice.

(Bereaved female)

Neighbours came to help, rice, sugar, coffee, and help looking after the corpse.

(Bereaved female)

The above type of community support reflects the findings of Hobfoll *et al*'s (2007) study into trauma interventions, which highlighted the need for interventions which emphasise self and collective efficacy, connectedness and hope.

Sub-theme: counselling and employment

The tragedy saw a number of women and children lose their husbands and fathers, respectively. The effects for this group of women were particularly sad and tragic as their loss extended across a number of areas: they lost not only their husband, the family's main breadwinner, but also their married status in Balinese society. The women bravely tried to cope and plan for the future of their family, with great pride and resilience. Resilience in this instance meant that the women displayed some signs of distress, but recovered enough from their initial symptoms to go about their daily lives and function at a reasonable level. Most of the women accepted their fate as part of the Hindu notion of *Karma* (Hobfoll *et al*, 2009; Norris *et al*, 2009).

One of the participants and her teenage son and daughter were devastated by the loss of their husband, father and breadwinner. Economically they struggled to survive and the woman was unable to buy her children clothes, mobile phones or shoes. She described the deep sadness she and her children felt. Fortunately, free counselling was available and the family received it once and sometimes twice a month for a year. Once a month she meets up with other widows who also lost their husbands in the tragedy. These support mechanisms have helped the family; however, an improved economic situation would continue the progress to a brighter future for all:

> It could convince me that I could survive and don't need to be sad all the time. From other widows we have the same destiny and . . . many more people have more bad destiny than me. If I could find a good job I will not be drowning in sorrow.
>
> (Bereaved female)

Another widow – aged 37 years, with three children aged 17, 11 and 8 years – described how she felt in 2002 shortly after she had received the news that her husband had been killed. In 2008, when the interview took place, this participant's outlook on life and personal circumstances had changed due to a number of support factors. A good family and community support network has given her and her family the vital support it needed. She has received money for school fees from YKIDS and also secured employment at a sewing co-operative set up for the women who lost their husbands in the bombing. All of this gave her 'the spirit to live again':

> I lost the family . . . breadwinner. I was sad, lost, don't know what to do, was empty and hollow. I must support three children but have not got a job and am sick. It was difficult to accept what happened. I lost the spirit of life because children made it hard. Don't know what to do as husband and car wrecked in the event. . . I can accept losing husband, can now bring up children, can continue with the future. Now lots of support from family and many parties [people]. I have friends and can work in the co-op although am feeling sick. I have spirit to live again. Thankful that kids got school because of YKIDS' help.
>
> (Bereaved female)

Reinforced resource 2: suggestions

Sub-theme: economic support

Participants in Bali were also keen to offer suggestions for support that may be helpful in similar circumstances. The issue of economic support was at the forefront of comments. The disruption to human capacity, in the form of livelihoods, was a regular discussion in all sections of this chapter. To help remedy their dire financial circumstances, victims suggested there was a need for job creation or money from the government to set up businesses.

It was noted that the government encouraged banks to be sympathetic to businesses, particularly with regard to late repayment of loans (hotel owner, personal communication, 2008). Other comments reflected the participants' need for continued health care and their anger at the perpetrators. Many wished for a safer future for Bali, with no more bombings. Overall the participants seemed to be expressing hope for the future of Bali and for themselves: an important part of the recovery process, as supported by the findings of Hobfoll *et al* (2007).

> Money for life support and a job for continuous family life.
>
> (Bereaved female)

A female participant who had been affected by the bombing wanted help from the government to start a business. She had asked (as did a number of the participants) if the victims in Perth got monetary support from the government. In Bali, the government helped with medical care initially, but after that phase it appears that the support ended. It was left to NGOs, friends, family members and neighbours to practically and financially support participants who were unable to return to work or who had lost a loved one in the bombing (as discussed above).

> The government in Bali (need to) provide help to set up new business, with financial support to set up [our] own business.
>
> (Injured female)

Sub-theme: no more bombings

A number of participants stated they wanted an end to bombings in Bali so that they and their families and friends could feel safe again, and so that tourists would return. This would lead to a return of economic stability for the island and an improved economy at macro and micro levels. More businesses would be created and existing businesses would feel more economically secure in continuing to employ their existing staff. Business sector confidence would subsequently increase and investment in new and existing businesses recommence. The jobs created would result in more families having economic stability, which all participants wanted. Other participants wanted the perpetrators severely punished and for tourists to return.

> If economics would be fine Bali would be safe. . . I need more medical and financial support. I don't like Amrozi, execute as soon as possible. . . I hope for a better future for Bali with no more bombs. I hope Bali could get back [the] trust of the world.
>
> (Injured female)

I hope no more bombs so a lot of tourist[s] will come to Bali so the salary will rise and [it will be] more easy to find a job. Why the people who did this till now haven't [been executed]?. . . If it not [happen] they could do anything they want.

(Wife of injured male)

The following participant felt that the community should also be more proactive in policing the activities of strangers in the community, to help avoid similar events:

I can't judge someone who create[s a] bomb, but their intellect is narrow-mind[ed] . . . to judge others. The banjar [type of community police] should be more community active, especially with people who come to Bali without any clear purpose.

(Injured male)

Social ecology

In this section, analysis of the data from the semi-structured interviews continues within the domain of social ecology, which is the social capital of a community and encompasses social relationships within families, peer groups, religious and cultural institutions and links with civic and political authorities (PWG, 2003). It is the links and connections with these groups which are often disrupted in complex emergencies such as terrorist attacks and natural disasters as family members are killed, go missing or are injured and vital infrastructure such as roads, telephone communications and businesses is damaged and destroyed. As these resources are disrupted, communities and their members respond and unite to support each other in a process of adjustment to the challenges they face. This process is called 'social bonding' and its effectiveness is an indicator of the resilience of the community (PWG, 2003). Figure 3.2 illustrates the disrupted and reinforced resources within the context of social ecology and is followed by a discussion of each theme, supported by relevant participant quotes.

Disrupted resource 1: effects

Sub-theme: children's psychological distress

Many of the Balinese victims were married with young children, and the children's emotional distress in the aftermath of the bombing was extensive. The children became secondary victims of the disaster as a number of them lived in the area with their parents and heard the bombs detonate and saw the burning buildings. To compound their trauma, in many instances one of their parents was injured in the bombing, and they could see for themselves the injuries and discomfort their parents were experiencing. In some cases, victims who had received extensive burns in the attack reported their children were quite distressed when they visited them in hospital, as their limbs or faces were initially quite swollen.

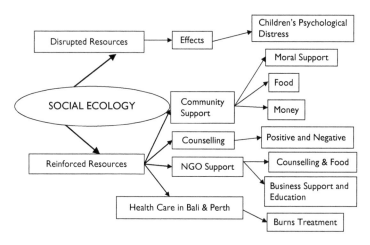

Figure 3.2 Social ecology – Bali

In addition, many of the participants and other informants in Bali reported that television and newspaper coverage of the attack was extremely graphic (personal communication, February 2008). A new television station had just commenced broadcasting in Bali when the attack occurred, and was on the scene and at the main hospital very soon after the attack. Anecdotal reports reveal that graphic and bloody scenes were filmed at the bombing site and the hospital, without any degree of censorship.

In some instances children's parents were not at home to censor their initial viewing of the event. These graphic scenes added to the children's considerable distress; it is now recognised that victims who were not directly exposed to critical incidents but who view them on television or in print may also present with some distress, as well as depression, nightmares and anxiety (Dougall *et al*, 2005; Park *et al*, 2008; Propper *et al*, 2007). The children's considerable distress and fear as a result of these factors is evident from their parents' descriptions (provided in chapter 7). In one instance the child was still afraid in 2008; another's distress continued for a further three years.

Reinforced resource 1: community support

Sub-themes: moral support, food and money

The economic effect on Bali and on individuals was difficult to assess. Many struggled to buy the basic necessities for life and to feed their families. As in Perth, the community members in Bali rallied to help individuals and families in the aftermath of the bombing. Many of the Balinese victims reported their gratitude for the moral and practical support they received in the form of donations of food and money from their family, friends and neighbours.

> There was no material support, just moral support. I feel the moral support was really useful for me because I look after the two of my children by myself.
>
> (Injured female)

> The head of the village gave me 50,000 IDR and neighbours and friends gave me moral support; they came to talk.
>
> (Injured female)

> My neighbour gave me noodles and rice. My neighbours visited my husband in hospital. Some of them gave money as well.
>
> (Wife of injured male)

Reinforced resource 2: counselling support

Sub-themes: positives and negatives

As in Perth, the primary victims and family members were offered counselling at Sanglah hospital by resident psychiatrists. Victims in Bali tended to have more contact with psychiatrists, while in Perth victims mostly saw counsellors and psychologists, with a few victims and family members referred to a psychiatrist. A number of participants were advised by their psychiatrist to pray to their god so they would feel comforted. The following respondent disclosed how her psychiatrist encouraged her to pray; this would be culturally and clinically appropriate here, as religion plays a very important part in the lives of most individuals in Bali.

> He suggests me to pray to the God. If I do believe in God everything will be fine.
>
> (Injured female, commenting on her psychiatrist's approach)

The psychiatrist in this instance revealed some personal details about his family. In this instance the disclosure may of been part of an approach that is favoured in the literature and termed 'compassionate witnessing', in which the therapist fosters a gentle, collaborative and respectful approach which, in the early stages of therapy, will reduce the likelihood of clients developing PTSD symptoms (Foa et al, 2005). On this occasion it seemed appropriate and reassuring for the participant.

> So I could feel confident to meet friends and not just stay alone in my room. He told me a nice story about his children and family, so I could feel better, so I could sleep.
>
> (Injured female, commenting on her psychiatrist's approach)

However, one of the male victims had mixed reactions to the counselling he had received and shared the single negative report given of the counselling offered in

Bali. His therapist had also suggested the participant should pray and revisit the scenes mentally. However, this request seemed to cause the participant some distress: he did not agree with the idea of mentally revisiting the scenes, as this upset him. He complied initially, then discontinued, as he found the action of visually revisiting his experiences very disturbing.

> They asked me to pray to the god and to take enough rest. They asked me to forget that moment [at first]. . . . the counsellor said 'don't forget the moment [when the bomb went off] and imagine it in detail', but when I tried it I feel like an unpleasant surprise. I didn't do it.
>
> (Injured male)

Reinforced resource 3: NGO support

Sub-theme: counselling and food

Bali received significant financial donations to aid victims and their families both within Bali and around the world (YKIP, 2007). All of the victims and family members interviewed had received financial support from a community organisation. The money was usually directed to an existing organisation such as Rotary, Bali Haiti, the Red Cross or a new organisation set up to serve a perceived need and help cope with the influx of money donated (YKIP, 2007). Basic necessities such as food and medicine were also donated and helped the victims and their family members to survive. This was a classic case of the Balinese and world community responding to share resources in response to the crisis.

> The Bali Haiti Foundation [NGO] gave me money and the John Fawcett Foundation [NGO] gave me medicine.
>
> (Injured male)

Sub-theme: Business support and education

The donated monies were also used to provide business support and education for affected victims. These stories indicate how the support of communities and community organisations was extremely helpful in the aftermath of the bombings as victims struggled to survive and support their families. As previously stated, there is no government unemployment benefit in Bali, and therefore the community and NGO support was not only useful – it was essential.

> Rotary supplied money and rice, Bali Haiti [NGO] foundation supplied medicines for the health of children and YKIDS [NGO] paid for the children's school fees.
>
> (Mother-in-law of deceased female)

Bali Haiti supplied money for rice and food for almost two years and YKIDS [paid] my daughter's school fees.

(Wife of injured male)

Reinforced resource 4: health care in Bali and Perth

Sub-theme: burns treatment

As with the victims from Perth, many of the victims from Bali received blast and burn injuries. Initially they received treatment at Sanglah hospital in Bali, and a number of the more severely injured who required specialised burns and hearing treatment were airlifted to Perth. As described by the participants, part of the treatment was paid for by the Balinese Red Cross and the Bali Haiti Foundation. In addition many of the specialists in Perth worked for no fee or for a lower than usual fee, although some charged the full price for their services (participant communication, 20 February 2008), The participants asked the researcher to thank the people of Australia who were involved in the care and expertise they experienced in Perth.

I got treatment at Sanglah for one month then in Oct 2002 I was treated at Perth for ear operations and cosmetic surgery.

(Injured female, who received
severe burns to her face and hearing damage)

In 2002, I had burns treatment at Sanglah hospital in ICU for three days and a burns operation. Seven days later I went to Perth for burns treatment. In May and July the next year I had further treatment in Perth.

(Injured male with severe burns)

In Dec 2002 I went to Perth for an eye operation paid for by Bali Haiti.

(Injured male with eye injuries)

Although the initial burn treatment was swift and efficient, a number of the burn victims required further treatment due to the thickening of their scars over the years, which caused restricted movement. For the first victim quoted above, this entailed two further trips to Perth, with all expenses paid, for further treatment.

Culture and values

This final section of the chapter presents analysis of the interview data within the domain of culture and values, which encompasses human rights, cultural values and beliefs that are disrupted in complex emergencies. These disruptions generate a sense of 'violation of human rights and an undermining of cultural values' (Strang and Ager, 2003, p. 3). The people of Bali struggled to understand why this

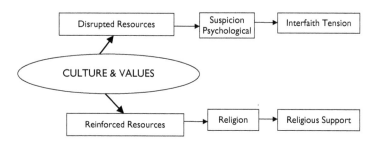

Figure 3.3 Culture and values – Bali

terrible event had occurred on their idyllic island. Many asked 'why are the Gods angry?' and 'what have we done to deserve this?'

As reflected in Figure 3.3 under the domain of culture and values, the interviews documented disrupted resources under the category of suspicion, which included interfaith tensions that occurred directly after the bombing. The reinforced resources documented religion as sustaining victims in the aftermath of the crisis. Each of these resources are further explained in detail below.

Disrupted resource 1: suspicion

Sub-theme: interfaith tension

Many of the participants were surprised and very disappointed by what had happened to 'their' Bali. They were confused and frightened and, in many cases, felt it was a sign they had done something wrong, in this life or a past life. To counteract these feelings, many people sought comfort in their religious beliefs and practices. The majority of participants were Hindu; they prayed and attended religious ceremonies.

For many others, the events of 2002 would leave them with a deep suspicion of Muslims, as the bombers who carried out the bombing were Muslims. The Muslim members of the community admitted to being angry and emotional, and many believed the bombers had misunderstood the religion of Islam. The Muslim participants deplored the attacks and their widespread ramifications for interfaith relationships in Bali. This sentiment was also expressed by non-Muslims, who reported a weakening of links with the Muslim community. The wider community in Bali firmly believed the bombings had been carried out by Muslims, and communities become suspicious of each other in the aftermath of the crisis. In this instance, the community suspicions were correct; the three men eventually convicted of and executed for the attack were Muslim.

The interfaith tensions are illustrated by the following participant, who explains that after the bombing he initially felt hate for Muslims, but this has now has dissipated because he believes the majority of the Muslim community also feel what the bombers did was wrong:

> I had a hate feeling. I don't feel it [hate] anymore because from other Muslim community they feel what the terrorist[s] did was wrong.
>
> (Injured male)

This participant, like most of the Balinese participants, endured economic hardship following the attack. He also explained how the image of the Muslim in Bali was (negatively) affected, as the perpetrators were believed to be Muslim:

> It reduced the economic [state of the country] and the image of Muslim[s] in the community.
>
> (Injured male)

The following Muslim participants questioned why the bombing occurred in Bali. The first asked why a Muslim group would carry out such an attack in a community which had a long-standing history of harmonious relationships between the various faiths. The second found it difficult to comprehend that fellow Muslims would knowingly target members of their own religious community:

> I wonder why it happened. I think the relationship among the religion[s] in Bali is really good. Why [did] one group [do] this?
>
> (Injured female)

> Why in Bali was there a bomb and I became a victim? I wonder who did it and didn't believe it was people from the same religion [as] me [who] did it.
>
> (Injured female)

Reinforced resource 1: religion

Sub-theme: religious support

Most of the participants from Bali were practising Hindus – the predominant religion on the island. The participants almost universally expressed religious belief and stated that religion and religious practices sustained them in the aftermath of the crisis. A smaller section of participants interviewed were Muslims who described how their religion had also supported them through difficult times. Interestingly, a number of participants who had not been practising their religion seemed to find some comfort in returning to prayer.

When faced with difficult life events it is not unusual for people to report that religion gives them comfort; recent research suggests there may be a link between post-traumatic growth and religion and/or spirituality following traumatic events (Wilson and Boden, 2008). The following participant, who was injured in the bombing, reveals that his religion was a comfort to him and had helped him come to an understanding of why he should have suffered such injuries.

> As a Hindu I think this is my *Karma*; I should accept it.
>
> (Injured male)

Others shared how their religion had been a significant source of support in the aftermath of the bombing:

> Religion helped me spiritually, without religion I feel terrible
>
> (Injured male)

> By praying to God there is a way. Yes we always pray so we are protected and shown direct[ion] out of the negative.
>
> (Injured Muslim victim)

> If there is not a God I think I [would have] died. It helped me a lot.
>
> (Injured female)

This victim believed he had been 'chosen by God' so he could improve his life and be a better person than he was before the bombing:

> God chose me to be special [to be a victim of the bombing] so I could improve your life and doing everything good.
>
> (Injured male)

One of two participants who changed faith after the bombing revealed that she had converted from the Muslim to Christian faith as a result of the counselling and support she had been proffered following the bombing:

> Most [of the counselling] came from the priest and two friends at church. When I was unconscious Jesus came to me. I change my religion from Muslim to Christian.
>
> (Injured female)

Summary

This chapter presented analysis of the interviews conducted with the Balinese primary and secondary-level victims, underpinned by the dimensions of human capacity, social ecology and culture and values. Many of the victims in Bali cited how their religion brought comfort to them during this difficult period of time. This has been observed in studies of other disasters, such as 9/11, when religiosity was observed to be a good predictor of lower levels of mental health issues and intrusive memories in victims. Changes – either a strengthening or lessening of religious beliefs – have also been observed in victims who had a high level of exposure to the 2004 Asian tsunami (Hussain *et al*, 2011).

Those victims who experienced a strengthening of their beliefs were thought to have used religion as a coping mechanism previously during a major life event. Overall an increase in religiosity seemed to have a beneficial effect, while a decline in religious beliefs appeared to adversely affect victims of the New Zealand earthquake (Sibley and Bulbulia, 2012). These associations have been noted across most religions (Bruno, 2011) and are worthy of further study as an important adjunct to our understanding of disasters and the many important factors that contribute to supporting victims.

Note

1 Hurricane Katrina was a Severe Category 3 storm which crossed the coast in 2005, flooding 80 per cent of New Orleans and causing severe damage in coastal areas in the Gulf of Mexico states of the USA; approximately 1,800 people died and thousands were left homeless.

References

Adams, L. M. (2007). Mental health needs of disaster volunteers: A plea for awareness. *Perspectives in Psychiatric Care, 43*(1), 52–55.

Adams, R. E., and Boscarino, J. A. (2005). Differences in mental health outcomes among whites, African Americans, and Hispanics following a community disaster. *Psychiatry, 68*(3), 250–266.

Agronick, G., Stueve, A., Vargo, S., and O'Donnell, L. (2007). New York City young adults' psychological reactions to 9/11: Findings from the Reach for Health longitudinal study. *American Journal of Community Psychology, 39*(12), 9–90.

Alexander, D. A. (2005). Early mental health intervention after disasters. *Advances in Psychiatric Treatment, 11*, 12–18.

Asian Development Bank (2003). *Asian Development Outlook 2003: Developing Asia: Risks and uncertainties*, 1–68. Retrieved 20 Aug 2014 from http://www.adb.org/Documents/Books/ADO/2003/part1_1-e.asp.

Badan Pusat Statistik (2009). *Statistics of Bali province*. Retrieved 20 Aug 2014 from http://bali.bps.go.id/tabeldetail.php?ed=51000412&od=4&rd=&id=4

Bali 123 (n.d.). *The history of Bali*. Retrieved 20 Aug 2014 from http://www.bali123.com/bali_history.htm

Bonanno, G. A., Galea, S., Bucciarelli, A., and Vlahov, D. (2007). What predicts psychological resilience after disaster? The role of demographics, resources, and life stress. *Journal of Consulting and Clinical Psychology, 75*(5), 671–682.

Boscarino, J. A., and Adams, R. E. (2007). PTSD onset and course following the World Trade Center disaster: Findings and implications for the future research. *Social Psychiatry and Psychiatric Epidemiology, 44*, 887–898. doi: 10.1007/s00127-009-0011-y

Brand, M. W., Kerby, D., Elledge, B., Burton, T., Coles, D., and Dunn, A. (2008). Public health's response: Citizens' thoughts on volunteering. *Disaster Prevention Management, 17*(1), 54–61.

Bride, B. E. (2007). Prevalence of secondary stress among social workers. *Social Worker*, 52(1), 63–70.

Brookes, G. (2010). The multilayered effects and support received by victims of the Bali bombings: A cross cultural study in Indonesia and Australia. Unpublished Doctor of Philosophy (PhD) Thesis. Curtin University, Perth, Western Australia.

Bruno, S. A. (2011). *Adjustment following natural disasters: The roles of trauma symptoms, religious coping, and locus of control.* Retrieved 20 Aug 2014 from ProQuest Dissertations and Theses, University of Houston, 91.

Buesnel, G. (2004). *All soldiers have nightmares.* Paper presented at the Australian Institute of Criminology Conference of Crime in Australia: International Connections. Melbourne. Retrieved 20 Aug 2014 from http://www.aic.gov.au/events

Cohen, R. (2002). Mental health services for victims of disasters. *World Psychiatry*, 1(3), 149–152.

Davis, J. L., Byrd, P., Rhudy, J. L., and Wright, D. C. (2007). Characteristics of chronic nightmares in a trauma-exposed treatment-seeking sample. *American Psychological Association*, 17(4), 187–198.

DiMaggio, C., Galea, S., and Li, G. (2009). Substance use and misuse in the aftermath of terrorism. A Bayesian meta-analysis. *Addiction*, 104, 894–904. Retrieved 20 Aug 2014 from http://hdl.handle.net/2027.42/. doi:10.3928/15394492-20091214-05.

Dougall, A. L., Hayward, M. C., and Baum, A. (2005). Media exposure to bioterrorism: Stress and the anthrax attacks. *Psychiatry: Interpersonal and Biological Processes*, 68(1), 28–42.

Edelhäuser, F. (2005). Religion in Bali. *Area-Striata*. Retrieved 20 Aug 2014 from http://area-striata.de/indonesia/religion.php

Fetter, J. (2005). Psychosocial responses to mass casualty terrorism: Guidelines for physicians. *Journal of Clinical Psychiatry*, 7(2), 49–52.

Foa, E. B., Cahill, S. P., Boscarino, J. A., Hobfoll, S. E., Lahad, M., McNally, R. J., and Solomon, Z. (2005). Social, psychological, and psychiatric interventions following terrorist attacks: Recommendations for practice and research. *Neuropsychopharmacology*, 30, 1806–1817.

Forbes, D., Wolfgang, B., Cooper, J., Creamer, M., and Barton, D. (2009). Post traumatic stress disorder. *Australian Family Physician*, 38(3), 106–111.

Giosan, C., Malta, L., Jayasinghe, N., Spielman, L., and Difede, J. (2009). Relationships between memory inconsistency for traumatic events following 9/11 and PTSD in disaster restoration workers. *Journal of Anxiety Disorders*, 23, 557–561.

Gregerson, M. B. (2007). Creativity enhances practitioners' resiliency and effectiveness after a hometown disaster. *Professional Psychology: Research and Practice*, 38(6), 596–602.

Hirschman, C., and Teerawichitchainan, B. (2003). Cultural and socioeconomic influences on divorce during modernization: Southeast Asia, 1940s to 1960s. *Population and Development Review*, 29(2), 215–253.

Hirst, W., Phelps, E. A., Buckner, R. L., Budson, A. E., Cuc, A., and Gabrieli, J. D. (2009). Long-term memory for the terrorist attack of September 11: Flashbulb memories, event memories, and the factors that influence their retention. *Journal of Experimental Psychology: General*, 138(2), 161–176.

Hobfoll, S. E., Watson, P., Bell, C. C., Bryant, R. A., Brymer, M. J., Friedman, M. J., Ursano, R. J. (2007). Five essential elements of immediate and mid-term mass trauma intervention: Empirical evidence. *Psychiatry*, 70(4), 283–315; discussion 316–369.

Retrieved 20 Aug 2014 from http://search.proquest.com/docview/220670681?
accountid=10382

Hobfoll, S. E., Palmeiri, P. A., Johnson, R. J., Canetti-Nisim, D., Hall, B. J., and Galea, S. (2009). Trajectories of resilience, resistance, and distress during ongoing terrorism: The case of Jews and Arabs in Israel. *Journal of Counselling and Clinical Psychology, 77*(1), 138–148.

Hobfoll, S. E., Watson, P., Bell, C. C., Bryant, R. A., Brymer, M. J., Friedman, M. J., and Ursano, R. J. (2007). Five essential elements of immediate and mid-term trauma intervention: Empirical evidence. *Psychiatry, 70*(4), 283–304.

Holmes, L. (2005). Marking the anniversary: Adolescents and September 11 healing process. *International Journal of Group Psychotherapy, 55*(3), 433–442.

Howe, L. (2006). *Terrorism in indirectly affected populations.* Paper presented at the Social Change in the 21st Century Conference at the Centre for Social Change Research: Queensland University of Technology.

Howe, L. (2001). *Hinduism and Hierarchy in Bali.* Oxford: James Currey.

Hussain, A., Weisaeth, L., and Heir, T. (2011). Changes in religious beliefs and the relation of religiosity to posttraumatic stress and life satisfaction after a natural disaster. *Social Psychiatry and Psychiatric Epidemiology, 46*(10), 1027–1032.

Jayarathne, S. S. (2014). Women's potential in dealing with natural disasters: A case study from Sri Lanka. *Asian Journal of Women's Studies, 20*(1), 125–136, 180.

Jayasinghe, N., Giosan, C., Evans, S., Spielman, L., and Difede, J. (2008). Anger and post traumatic stress disorder in disaster relief workers exposed to the September 11, 2001 World Trade Center disaster: One-year follow-up study. *Journal of Nervous and Mental Disease, 196*(11), 844–856.

Jones, G. W., and Gubhaju, B. (2008). *Trends in age at marriage in the provinces of Indonesia.* Asia Research Institute: Working Paper Series No 105. Retrieved 20 Aug 2014 from http://www.ari.nus.edu.sg/docs/wps/wps08_105.pdf

Kinsel, J., and Thomasgard, M. (2008). In their own words: The 9/11 disaster child care providers. *Families, Systems and Health, 26*(1), 44–57.

Lawyer, S. R., Resnick, H. S., Galea, S., Ahern, J., Kilpatrick, D. G., and Vlahov, D. (2006). Predictors of peritraumatic reactions and PTSD following the September 11th terrorist attacks. *Psychiatry: Interpersonal and Biological Processes, 69*(2), 130–141.

Mansdorf, I. J. (2008). Psychological intervention following terrorist attacks. *British Medical Bulletin, 88*(1), 7–22.

McCaslin, S. E., Jacobs, G. A., Meyer, D. L., Johnson-Jimenez, E., Metzler, T. J., and Marmar, C. R. (2005). How does negative change following disaster response impact distress among Red Cross responders? *Professional Psychology: Research and Practice, 36*(3), 246–253.

MacGeorge, E. L., Samter, W., Feng, B., Gillihan, S. J., and Graves, A. R. (2004). Stress, social support, and health among college students after September 11, 2001. *Journal of College Student Development, 45*(6), 655–668.

Meisenhelder, J. B., and Marcum, J. P. (2009). Terrorism, post-traumatic Stress, coping strategies, and spiritual outcomes. *Journal of Religion and Health, 48*(1), 46–57.

Miller, L. (2004). Psychotherapeutic interventions for survivors of terrorism. *American Journal of Psychotherapy, 58*(1), 1–16.

Mitka, M. (2008). PTSD prevalence still high for persons living near World Trade Center attacks. *JAMA, 300*(7), 779.

Moore, R. S., Cunradi, C. B., and Ames, G. M. (2004). Did substance use change after September 11th? An analysis of a military cohort. *Military Medicine, 169*(10), 829–832.

Moscardino, U., Scrimin, S., Capello, F., and Altoe, G. (2010). Social support, sense of community, collective values, and depressive symptoms in adolescent survivors of the 2004 Beslan terrorist attack. *Social Science and Medicine, 70,* 27–34.

Muñoz, M., Crespo, M., Pérez-Santos, E., and Vázquez, J. J. (2004). We were all wounded on March 11 in Madrid: Immediate psychological effects and interventions. *European Psychologist, 9*(4), 278–280.

National Center for PTSD: US Department of Veterans Affairs (2009). *The PILOTS database.* Retrieved 20 Aug 2014 from http://www.ptsd.va.gov/professional/pilots-database/pilots-db.asp

Neria, Y., Olfson, M., Gameroff, M. J., Wickramaratne, P., Gross, R., and Pilowsky, D. (2008). The mental health consequences of disaster-related loss: Findings from primary care one year after the 9/11 terrorist attacks. *Psychiatry, 71*(4), 339–348.

Norris, F. H., Tracy, M., and Galea, S. (2009). Looking for resilience: Understanding the longitudinal trajectories of responses to stress. *Social Science and Medicine, 68,* 2190–2198.

Orth, U., Cahill, S. P., Foa, E. B., and Maercker, A. (2008). Anger and posttraumatic stress disorder symptoms in crime victims: A longitudinal analysis. *Journal of Consulting and Clinical Psychology, 76*(2), 208–218.

Osinubi, O. Y., Gandhi, S. K., Ohman-Strickland, P., Boglarsky, C., Fiedler, N., Kipen, H., and Robson, M. (2008). Organisational factors and office workers health after the World Trade Center terrorist attacks: Long term physical symptoms, psychological distress, and work productivity. *Journal of Occupational Environmental Medicine. 50,* 112–125.

Park, C. L., Aldwin, C. M., Fenster, J. R., and Snyder, L. B. (2008). Pathways to posttraumatic growth versus posttraumatic stress: Coping and emotional reactions following the September 11, 2001, terrorist attacks. *American Journal of Orthopsychiatry, 78*(3), 300–312.

Pedersen, L. (2009). *Keeping Bali strong? Inside Indonesia 95.* Retrieved 20 Aug 2014 from http://www.insideindonesia.org/edition-95/keeping-bali-strong

Perina, K. (2002). Hot on the trail of flashbulb memory. *Psychology Today, March 2002.* Retrieved 20 Aug 2014 from http://www.psychologytoday.com/articles/200203/hot-the-trail-flashbulb-memory

Pfeffer, C. R., Altemus, H., Heo, M., and Jiang, M. (2009). Salivary cortisol and psychopathology in adults bereaved by the September 11, 2001 terror attacks. *International Journal of Psychiatry in Medicine, 39*(3), 215–216.

Propper, R. E., Stickgold, R., Keeley, R., and Christman, S. D. (2007). Is television traumatic? Dreams, stress, and media exposure in the aftermath of September 11, 2001. *Psychological Science, 18*(4), 334–340.

Psychosocial Working Group (PWG) (2003). *Psychosocial intervention in complex emergencies: A framework for practice.* Working Paper, Centre for International Health Studies, Queen Margaret University, Edinburgh.

Pulido, M. L. (2007). In their words: Secondary traumatic stress in social workers responding to the 9/11 terrorist attacks in New York. *Social Work, 52*(3), 279–281.

Rao, K. (2006). Psychosocial support in disaster-affected communities. *International Review of Psychiatry, 18*(6), 501–505. doi:1237467351.

Richman, J. A., Cloninger, L., and Rospenda, K. M. (2008). Macrolevel stressors, terrorism, and mental health outcomes: Broadening the stress paradigm. *American Journal of Public Health, 98*(2), S113–S119.

Saul, B. (2008). Defining terrorism in international law. *European Law Journal, 14*(4), 509–511.

Shalev, A. Y., Tuval, R., Frenkiel-Fishman, S., Hadar, H., and Eth, S. (2006). Psychological responses to continuous terror: A study of two communities in Israel. *American Journal of Psychiatry, 163*(4), 667–673.

Sibley, C. G., and Bulbulia, J. (2012). Faith after an earthquake: A longitudinal study of religion and perceived health before and after the 2011 Christchurch, New Zealand earthquake. *PLoS One, 7*(12). doi:http://dx.doi.org/10.1371/journal.pone.0049648

Steffen, S. L., and Fothergill, A. (2009). 9/11 volunteerism: A pathway to personal healing and community engagement. *The Social Science Journal, 46*(1), 29–46.

Steury, S., Spencer, S., and Parkinson, G. W. (2004). The social context of recovery. *Psychiatry: Interpersonal and Biological Processes, 67*(2), 158–163.

Strang, A. B., and Ager, A. (2003). Psychosocial interventions: Some key issues facing practitioners. *Intervention, 3*(1), 2–12.

Swygard, H., and Stafford, R. E. (2009). Effects on health of volunteers deployed during a disaster. *The American Surgeon, 75*(9), 747–753.

Taylor, A. J. (1990). A pattern of disasters and victims. *Disasters, 14*(4), 291–300.

Tuchner, M., Meiner, Z., Parush, S., and Hartman-Maeir, A. (2010). Relationships between sequelae of injury, participation, and quality of life in survivors of terrorist attacks. *OTJR: Occupation, Participation and Health, 30*(1), 29–36.

Van Ommeren, M., Saxena, S., and Saraceno, B. (2005). Mental and social health during and after acute emergencies: Emerging consensus. *Bulletin of the World Health Organisation, 83*(1), 71–76.

Vijaykumar, L., Thara, R., John, S., and Chellappa, S. (2006). Psychosocial intervention after tsunami in Tamil Nadu, India. *International Review of Psychiatry, 18*(3), 225–231.

Vlahov, D., Galea, S., Ahern, J., Rudenstine, S., Resnick, H., and Kilpatrick, D. (2006). Alcohol drinking problems among New York City residents after the September 11 terrorist attacks. *Substance Use and Misuse, 41*(9), 1295–1311.

Walsh, F. (2007). Traumatic loss and major disasters: Strengthening family and community resilience. *Family Process, 46*(2), 207–227.

Watchorn, J. H. (2001). *Surviving Port Arthur: the role of dissociation in the impact of psychological trauma and its implications for the process of recovery* (Doctoral dissertation). Retrieved 20 Aug 2014 from http://eprints.utas.edu.au/1271/. (ID Code: 1271).

Wilson, J. T., and Boden, J. M. (2008). The effects of personality, social support and religiosity on posttraumatic growth. *The Australasian Journal of Disaster and Trauma Studies, 1*, 1–17.

Wilson, N., d'Ardenne, P., Scott, C., Fine, H., and Priebe, S. (2012). Survivors of the London bombings with PTSD: A qualitative study of their accounts during CBT treatment. *Traumatology, 18*(2), 75–84.

Women's Refugee Commission (2014). Retrieved 20 Aug 2014 from http://womens refugeecommission.org/programs/reproductive-health/disaster-risk-reduction

Yehudi, R., and Hyman, S. (2005). The impact of terrorism on brain and behaviour: What we know and what we need to know. *Neuropsychopharmacology, 30*(10), 1773–1780. Retrieved 20 Aug 2014 from http://www.dwamusa.com/impact_of_terrorism_on_brain.htm

YKIP (2007). *YKIP's Journey: The first five years.* Bali, Indonesia: Annika Linden Foundation and Reset.

Chapter 4

The effects on victims in Perth

Introduction

This chapter presents the effects on the primary (PLV) and secondary-level victims (SLV) from the Perth suburb of Kingsley. First, a socio-demographic profile of the participants is presented; this is followed by a presentation of the interview data that came from the semi-structured interviews, which gives voice to the personal experiences of primary and secondary-level victims.

Socio-demographic profiles of the participants: Perth

The following section presents an analysis of the demographic data collected from PLV and SLV participants in Perth and reveals the varying socio-economic statuses, living conditions and educational levels of participants in Perth.

Age and gender

The lower age limit for participation in this study was 18 years. The PLV age groupings were split between the ages of 19–24 years (n = 1), 25–30 years (n = 1), 31–36 years (n = 1) and 37–42 years (n = 1) (Table 4.1). The group that travelled to Bali was a mixture of players from Kingsley Football Club, coaching staff and the players' friends, hence the mix of age groups. The oldest person to go on the trip was a 41-year-old member of the club's support team. He was one of the most badly injured members of the team and was airlifted to Darwin for intensive emergency treatment. The PLV were all male (as one would expect in an Australian Rules Football team from Perth).

Of the five participants in the SLV group, one participant was in the 25–30 years age grouping, half of the remainder were in the 43–48 years age grouping (n = 2) and two were in the 49–54 years age grouping (n = 2); three were female and two were male (Table 4.2). They were mainly parents of participants who had been injured or killed, hence the older age grouping, at 43–54 years (n = 4). Three of the participants were on the Kingsley Football Club committee and a fourth was the husband of a committee member. All SLV participants were closely connected to the football club, either as past players or as parents of football players who had been killed or injured in the bombing.

Marital status

A higher proportion of the five SLV participants (three) were married; one participant was divorced, and one was single. In Perth, the pattern of divorce is presently declining. This decline in the rate of divorce is thought to be due to the older age of first marriage (32.1 years for males, 29.5 years for females) and the fact that 75 per cent of couples cohabit before marriage (Australian Government Australian Institute of Family Studies, 2008). In the PLV group, two were in a de facto relationship, one was married and one was single.

Education

Education in Western Australia, as in all the other states and territories of Australia, is compulsory and is provided free by the government in each state. Children must attend school or be home-schooled from the age of 5 years until the end of the year in which they turn 16 (Australian Government, n.d.). Of the PLV group, all had attended primary and secondary school, with one having also attended tertiary education. In the SLV group all attended primary and secondary schooling and one attended tertiary education.

Income

Of the PLV, three declared a regular income and one participant declined to give their income. Their monthly incomes ranged from $2,900 to $5,600. The minimum wage set in Western Australia is $2,229.60 per month (West Australian Industrial Relations Commission, 2007) and the monthly income of all PLV participants was above this minimum wage. The SLVs' monthly income ranged from $14,000 per month at the highest to $1,350 at the lowest, for a part-time worker.

Employment

In terms of employment, all PLVs were employed prior to the Bali bombing (n = 4, 100% per cent, as were all of the SLVS (n = 5, 100 per cent). Post-bombing and at the time of interview in 2008, all the participants from Perth were employed in a full-time or part-time capacity (n = 9, 100 per cent). Perth is a rich state, with mineral resources contributing to the state's positive wealth and employment statistics (Australian Institute of Company Directors, 2007). Perth's unemployment rate was a low 3.4 per cent in 2008, despite the beginnings of the economic downturn (Australian Bureau of Statistics, 2008). The demographics of PLV in Perth is presented in Tables 4.1 and 4.2 (see over).

Table 4.1 Demographic characteristics of primary-level victims – Perth

Demographic and descriptive variables	Total Participants n = 4
Age	
19–24 years	1
25–30 years	1
31–36 years	1
37–42 years	1
Gender	
Female	0
Male	4
Marital Status	
De facto	2
Married	1
Single	1
Education	
Primary	4
Secondary	4
Tertiary	1
Employment	
Employed	4
Unemployed	0
Monthly Income	
A$4,000–6,000	1
A$3,000–4,000	1
A$2,000–3,000	1
Did not respond	1

Religion

None of the PLV group identified with any religion. Of the five SLV participants, all stated they were Christian. A number of the SLV participants did state that they prayed or turned to their religion to help cope with the difficulties they were facing: this is not unusual in times of crisis, when religion becomes a coping mechanism for many people (Ai *et al*, 2005).

Forms of support

The PLVs and SLVs received medical, counselling and spiritual and community support from a number of sources in varying amounts (Table 4.3). Of the PLV group, one received support from two sources, namely counselling and community support. Two received support from three sources: medical, counselling and community support. The other received support from four sources, namely medical, counselling, community and religious support. Of the SLV participants, three received support in the form of counselling, two in the form of counselling and community support and one in the form of medical, counselling, community and

Table 4.2 Demographic characteristics of secondary-level victims – Perth

Demographic and descriptive variables	Total Participants n = 5
Age	
25–30 years	1
43–48 years	2
49–54 years	2
Gender	
Female	3
Male	2
Marital Status	
Married	3
Divorced	1
Single	1
Religion	
Christian	5
Education	
Primary	5
Secondary	5
Tertiary	1
Employment	
Employed	5
Unemployed	0
Monthly Income	
A$12,000–14,000	1
A$4,000–6,000	1
A$2,000–4,000	1
A$1,000–2,000	1
Did not respond	1

Table 4.3 Forms of support – Perth

	Medical	Counselling	Community	Spiritual
PLVs	2	3	3	1
SLVs	1	6	3	1

religious support. For the SLV participants, counselling was the most popular form of support. From the contact the researcher had with the parents of injured players, it appeared that most initially sought counselling support in order to gain information to enable them to understand how to best support their injured or distressed family members.

The PLVs described how they were provided money to attend to bills, buy food and purchase suits to attend funerals, as well as the extensive emotional support they received from the Red Cross, volunteer psychologists, family friends and the pastor from their local church. The SLV participants described a similar mix of support from a number of government agencies, the Red Cross, family, friends and even people they hardly knew.

Summary

In Perth, none of the participants were living below the poverty line; any whose wage was below the minimum had a partner who was also working and whose income was not taken into account in this study. All had attended school up to secondary level (100%), and were employed either full time or part time by choice. In both groups the participants were provided a relatively high level of support from multiple sources, including financial, counselling, community, medical, and religious.

Analysis of interview data: Perth

The terms disrupted and reinforced resources were again used to organise and analyse the data using the psychosocial framework of human capacity, social ecology and culture and values. (Disrupted and reinforced resources are explained in greater depth in chapters 3 and 6.) The participants' accounts of their experiences formed important and unique insights into their experiences of the Bali bombing. The analysis commences within the domain of human capacity.

Human capacity

This section, which explores the element of human capacity, commences with a description of the three main categories of disrupted resources that emerged from the data and concludes with an analysis of the two categories of reinforced resources depicted diagrammatically in Figure 4.1.

The primary and secondary-level victims interviewed were all connected to Kingsley Football Club, in the northern suburbs of Perth. The participants describe their story and how their lives and resources were disrupted by the bombing. They also describe how resources within their families and community helped them in many different ways in the days and months following the bombing. Their stories catalogue not only the negative aspects of the bombing but also the many positive factors they experienced. While similarities can be identified in a number of the stories and the victims were involved in the same tragic event, it is important to highlight that their individual stories are unique and personal to each participant.

As reflected in Figure 4.1, the domain of human capacity draws on the concepts of *reinforced* and *disrupted* resources used to underpin the interview analysis. The interviews revealed disrupted resources under the categories of effects (psychological, physical and emotional), behaviours (risk-taking) and reactions

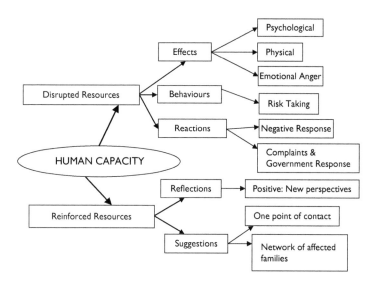

Figure 4.1 Human capacity – Perth

(negative responses and complaints). Reinforced resources revealed the themes of reflections (having positive and new perspectives) and suggestions (having one point of contact and forming a network of affected families). Each of these resources are further explained in detail below.

Disrupted resource 1: effects

Sub-theme: psychological effects

A number of the injured members of Kingsley Football Club graphically described the effect the bombing had on their lives. Having begun as happy tourists celebrating their end-of-season football final, they became victims of a terrorist attack (Davis *et al*, 2007). In the initial period following the bombing, the young participants from Kingsley Football Club described their confusion regarding what had happened, and suffering nightmares and a chronic lack of sleep – which is a normal reaction to a very abnormal experience (Meisenhelder and Marcum, 2009), and which would eventually dissipate.

As a result of their shared experiences, the young men felt a great need to be in contact with each other, would sleep with their mobile phones under their pillows and would contact each other for mutual support when still awake late at night or in the early hours of the morning. This social bonding of the young men through a traumatic shared event was an important factor in 2002, and for some it continues to the present day. Social bonding and mutual support was an important part of their psychosocial recovery. For some participants, lack of sleep and nightmares continued for a year after the event:

> I think it stopped my normal world almost totally. The hardest thing was dealing with the nightmares and lack of sleep.
>
> (Injured male, KAFC)

> For 12 months I had frequent nightmares. I would startle if there was a loud noise or a car backfired.
>
> (Injured male, KAFC)

> It was fairly catastrophic; it was gut-wrenching horrible.
>
> (Injured male, KAFC)

Sub-theme: ongoing psychological impacts

In 2008, six years after the bombings, none of the victims interviewed were receiving psychological interventions or counselling support, yet the ongoing emotional impact of the bombing was being described in detail by a number of victims across all levels. This occurred across the spectrum of primary-level victims, who were in or around the vicinity of the Sari club or Paddy's bar on that fateful night, to secondary-level family members who lost a loved one in the bombing or family members and friends who supported the injured victims when they returned home to Perth. One injured male participant continues to have nightmares and recognises that the events of the bombing are still with him:

> I watched a movie about a year ago called 'Ladder 49' and at the end it is just a bloke in a building with fire going around. I didn't think anything about it at the time until I woke up in the middle of the night with a nightmare. It's still in the back of my mind and things trigger it off.
>
> (Injured male, KAFC)

A friend of a deceased victim indicated he was grateful to be given the time and space to talk about his feelings. This participant described how he is unable to share his thoughts and inner feelings with anyone, and as a result tries to 'hold it all in' in an effort to protect his family members and friends, who he believes want him to move on and stop discussing the events:

> I still get upset over it. My mum says you have to get over it. I don't really understand what that means. . .
>
> (Friend of deceased male, KAFC)

In an attempt to cope with the enormity of what they have experienced, victims of trauma will sometimes display a process of denial and suppression which is termed adaptive disassociation (Watchorn, 2001). The following victim vividly described the suppression of his emotions:

> Compassion, sincerity and emotion – I don't really have them. Things don't get to me. Well they do, but not in a personal manner. . . . I've suppressed a lot of things.
>
> (Member, KAFC)

Terrorist attacks, which produce high levels of casualties "are shocking and dramatic and are likely to evoke strong emotions" (Blanchette *et al*, 2007, p. 49) in the civilian population who are targeted in the attacks. Within contemporary psychology, there is a trend towards 'positive psychology' (Duckworth *et al*, 2005; Linley *et al*, 2006) as the discipline attempts to move towards a more flexible understanding of the range of reactions victims may demonstrate in their response to difficult and traumatic life events (Linley *et al*, 2006). The initial post-event symptoms, such as shock, numbness and despair, are normal reactions to very abnormal circumstances (Rao, 2006, p. 506).

Sub-theme: physical effects

Many of the victims were evacuated to Perth with physical injuries received in the bombing. Two of the injured survivors were air-lifted to the Eastern States with life-threatening injuries, while seven remained in Bali with injuries consistent with the detonation of a suicide bomb. They reported primary injuries caused by exposure to the blast wave such as hearing damage. They also experienced injuries such as lacerations, back and shoulder damage, severe bruising and splinters of glass and wood throughout the body, which were likely caused as a result of flying objects energised by the wind blast, and miscellaneous injuries such as burns caused by the fire which occurred in the aftermath of the explosion (Moore, 2006). The injuries disrupted both physical and psychological aspects of their health and reduced their ability to work and interrelate in their usual capacity within the community.

Commonly, the young men minimised the extent of the injuries they had received. In the aftermath of the attack they appeared to ignore the pain from their burns and other injuries to search for their seven missing friends over a number of days. From the outset, those who had survived vowed to bring their friends back home to Perth, alive or deceased. The day after the bombing, they organised a search for their missing friends in hospitals, hotels and the morgue in Bali. They searched patient lists and photographic records of the dead and injured, and looked at numerous corpses in the morgue. This type of behaviour is consistent with the 'rescue phase' of a disaster, when altruism is at its highest and people who have been injured themselves take part in relief work (Rao, 2006).

Well physically there was a bit burnt here and there. . .
(Injured male, KAFC, who sustained burns to his arm and back)

I got a bit of a sore back; I got a few bruises at the top of my legs and a few splinters, and glass in my head from the initial blast, but nothing really.
(Injured male, KAFC)

At the time I still had a big piece of metal stuck in my shoulder blade that I was forced [by the other players] to get removed, because I didn't care about it.
(Injured male, KAFC, who waited until three days after the event to have treatment in Bali)

Sub-theme: emotional effects

At the time of their interviews, the young football players reported a range of emotions, with anger being the most frequent. The effects of the bombing were still being experienced and described in detail six years following the bombing. One young male player reported the need to attend the trial of the bombers in Bali. He described wanting to confront 'his demons', and afterwards reported 'feeling better' for attending the trial. Anger, particularly towards the perpetrators of an attack, is not an unusual emotion for victims of an attack to display or report (Miller, 2004). This following young man's anger may be a necessary outlet for his emotions and lead to eventual achievement of emotional stability and growth (Park et al, 2008):

There is still a bit of anger there for sure. I went to the initial trials to look Amrosi in the face and I felt better for that, as he is only a little bastard. I was angry and [am] still angry they did it.
(Injured male, KAFC)

One of the friends of a young man killed in the bombing revealed he often visits the graveyard where a number of his friends are buried. He goes when he feels emotions ranging from anger to sadness 'building up' and 'overflowing', and reports feeling calmer when he has been to the graveyard. As previously discussed, there is no rulebook or linear progression in grief or distress, particularly after a traumatic event. People will move in and out of grief as various anniversaries, birthdays and events remind them of that time in their lives. This young man was able to release his emotions in what he felt was a safe and significant venue where he could talk to his friends and cry and feel no one would judge him:

Late last year [2007] it affected me and it felt like it built up and overflowed and I went down to Pinnaroo [local graveyard] and sat down for a bit.
(Friend of victim, KAFC)

The following participant describes how the angry feelings he has regarding the bombing will often be displaced when he is angry and upset about something else. In psychological terms this is termed displaced anger; the participant is unable to lose or channel his anger at the perpetrators and will displace it when something unrelated to the attack triggers his anger.

> I think the anger comes out if I am upset about another situation.
>
> (Injured male, KAFC)

Disrupted resource 2: behaviours

Sub-theme: risk-taking behaviours

Over-indulgence, particularly with regard to alcohol, was a common coping mechanism for many of the young victims, as was the use of illicit drugs. Risk-taking behaviours, increased alcohol consumption or illicit drug use following trauma are not unusual for young males who have been exposed to life-threatening traumatic events (Moore *et al*, 2004; Vlahov *et al*, 2006). The young males who had been directly affected by the bombing, and some of their fathers, appeared to gravitate to the local tavern, which became a regular gathering point in the aftermath of the bombing and the six funerals of their mates in Perth.

Overall, the young men reported a loss of resources within both the physical and mental health spheres. Due to burns and other injuries most were unable to work for some months after the bombing, which meant their livelihoods were disrupted. This resulted in a disconnection with their work, their work colleagues and their community. Ultimately having no choice but to stay at home to allow their physical and psychological wounds to heal appeared to produce a reduced sense of control over their lives. The boredom, lack of connection with their work and work colleagues and lack of normal routine which they reported may be among the reasons why a number of the injured reported using copious amounts of alcohol and/or various amounts of illicit drugs in the aftermath of the bombing. A participant describes being in the pub with his friends from the KAFC. It seemed the group camaraderie and alcohol helped him and others cope with the enormity of what had happened:

> I spent a month solidly at the [. . .] tavern and I spent so much money. It was the best form of help I could have. It wasn't just alcohol-fuelled emotions; it was stuff that needed to come out. You'd walk out the front [of the tavern and] have a cry, ten boys would come outside and cry with you, you'd all have a laugh and walk in there and be fine again.
>
> (Injured male, KAFC)

This participant was using illicit drugs as a form of self-medication, which also enabled him to cope:

> My thing was I used illicit drugs to help get me through it. The way I looked at it, it was taking my mind off things and putting a smile on my face.
>
> (Injured male, KAFC)

Another participant also admitted he was self-medicating. It seemed he was unable to talk to his close family members about his experiences, so he joined in with his mates and drank copious amounts of alcohol:

> I had my mates. I recognised I was self-medicating with alcohol. I've never been able to talk to my parents about it. I have talked to my brothers about once or twice in the last five years about it.
>
> (Friend of deceased male, KAFC)

Disrupted resource 3: responses

Sub-theme: negative reactions

The impact of terrorist attacks is multifaceted and not limited to the people or the communities directly affected. Knowing someone who was killed or injured in a terrorist attack has been documented to increase the risk of developing physical and psychological symptoms such as those listed below. The victims of the Bali attack, their close family members and their friends described vivid reactions which ranged from entering coping mode to numbness and shock, or acting as if nothing had happened. As previously stated, this is termed 'adaptive disassociation', and it is one means by which some people will attempt to cope with an extremely difficult situation (Watchorn, 2001). Within the domain of human capacity, the participants reported many interruptions and challenges to their physical and mental well-being throughout the crisis. A participant who was a close friend of a missing, presumed deceased, victim described his reaction on the day after the bombing:

> The first day I was pretty casual about it. I was actually pretty clinical about it all. I was like, information is going to start coming in so I'll get all the boys together.
>
> (Friend of deceased male, KAFC)

Another victim described the dazed state he entered in the first few days, which enabled him to cope in the best way he could:

> I just closed up, didn't really say anything. I spent three to four days not knowing anyone. . . . so I just jumped in my car and left [when back in Perth].

I don't know where I went. I was gone for a while. I wanted to avoid it, not accept it I suppose.

(Friend of injured male, KAFC)

This participant vividly described his numbness and 'cutting off' of emotions during the many funerals he attended in the aftermath:

The emotion didn't really hit in, well it did for the extreme parts but it didn't hit in until we got back home. I think the shock covered everything for about a fortnight . . . when I went to about 12 or 15 funerals within three months, I felt no sadness at all. . . . It's just not real. I'm still waiting. It's probably going to hit me in 10 or 15 years' time.

(Injured male, KAFC)

In one of the longest interviews undertaken during this study, a mother described her thoughts and reactions at a very difficult time of loss and tragedy, and her grief over the loss of a precious son. She described in detail her daughter's confusion and emotional pain with great clarity, dignity and composure. As this was a new, over-whelming and tumultuous experience, it is understandable that individuals would struggle with their emotions, such as grief and disbelief. Grief is a very individual emotion and two people in a household may react quite differently. There is no right or wrong – just what is right, or feels right, for them at that time.

Feeling numb, reacting as if nothing had happened, or feeling dazed and con-fused can all be categorised as coping mechanisms that enable people to cope with trauma (Reosenthal, cited by Holmes, 2005, p. 434). The following partic-ipant quotes clearly illustrate this mechanism. This participant explained that she had two children and outlined how she and her daughter reacted on hearing the news her son had been killed:

I went into coping mode immediately. . . . I remained like that for about three months basically . . . [her daughter] was totally dazed, she had no idea. She was confused and lost.

(Mother 1)

The researcher also interviewed a number of women from the same football club whose sons had been injured in the bombing. They outlined how their sons and daughters in Perth had reacted to the news their sibling had been injured in the bombing. These descriptions are similar to the reaction of the young woman above: they went into a 'zombie-like' state of shock, numbness and disbelief.

My youngest son sort of walked around as if all was OK.

(Mother 2)

. . . went into. . . like a zombie mode. My son . . . completely went into denial.

(Mother 3)

Sub-theme: complaints and government response

A common theme among participants was their perception of the government's slow response in the initial phase of the crisis. It is important to note that a number of participants also stated that the government response was excellent once things 'got going'. All comments and suggestions were provided by participants in a constructive way and the aim was genuinely to improve the situation for others if a similar event were to ever occur again and impact Australian citizens.

> This is why I think it's great you're doing this. I didn't know who to talk to about this stuff. I felt that something needed to be done. That plane took an awful long time from Australia to get to Bali to get our people back. . . . I thought our planes didn't get through quick enough. We've got to stop the complacency; that's my biggest thing. They [the government] were way too slow.
>
> (Mother of deceased male, KAFC)

> The government were very slow. They were very good once they got motivated. We should have had somewhere to go; we should have had an official to talk to as next of kin, family; we should have had something. We should not have had to initiate it ourselves Monday, and I don't think it should happen again. There should be a quicker response to that sort of disaster. . .
>
> (Mother of injured male, KAFC)

> I would have liked official notification as soon as I could, even the following day; someone officially to say what happened.
>
> (Mother of injured male, KAFC)

Reinforced resource 1: reflections

Sub-theme: positives and new perspectives

As previously reported, just as resources can be disrupted by traumatic events, there are resources inherent within the wider community that can be reinforced and used to support victims. For many, the events of 12 October 2002 were life-changing, and a number of the participants reported they gained new perspectives on what was relevant, significant and important in life. For one victim in particular, this new perspective means he gets less upset at everyday events. Now he does not get angry at small, irrelevant things, whereas previously he would have reacted differently. This type of reflection is not unusual following a traumatic experience, as many victims strive to make greater meaning out of the experience. The search for deeper meaning, focusing on the positive following traumatic events, is thought to be an important coping mechanism and an indicator of personal resilience (Tatar and Amram, 2007).

I still find things like work irrelevant to life, when you sort of learn lessons like this; you sort of realise what is really important. . . I think it's the only way otherwise I'd still be in a pub drowning my sorrows. . . I just tried training myself to get some positives out of it.

(Injured male, KAFC)

For me it's given me a new perspective and helped me to grow. I definitely have changed in the last five years with outlooks into certain social and political issues. . . I really was really upset and [now] it takes a lot more than road rage to get me upset.

(Friend of deceased male, KAFC)

Reinforced resource 2: suggestions

Sub-theme: one point of contact

Participants were very willing to comment on strategies that might be useful in the event of a future disaster involving Australians or people from other nations. They were keen to propose suggestions in the hope that something good would evolve out of this terrible event. On their return to Perth, most of the injured required medical assessment, counselling and financial support from agencies such as Centrelink, the government social support agency which delivers a range of support services – including counselling and financial help – for those in need and is now part of the human service portfolio of the Department of Human Services; the Australian Red Cross in Western Australia, and their general practitioners (GPs).

For some this meant queuing at Centrelink, or waiting in a GP's waiting room, and a number of the victims noted the further distress caused by having to retell their story many times. The mother of one of the injured victims suggested reducing this distress by allocating a building or venue from the outset in which all important contacts, such as Centrelink, counsellors and doctors, were available 24/7 for the returning victims.

Some of the boys were a bit agro that they had to keep explaining. Every time you went to Centrelink you'd get someone different. You don't have to explain to a thousand different people. Later on they could branch out but initially there should have been one point of contact.

(Mother of injured male, KAFC)

Sub-theme: network for affected families

One participant felt that it would be useful to create a network for those who had been affected by the bombing so that families could support each other, especially those who had little or no family support of their own. An injured male reflected on the fact that the injured young men at the football club had a large network of support around them. He felt concerned for the other families who had people injured or killed in the bombing and did not have a close support network around them:

> My main concern and always has been for the families that were on their own. So I think there should be a bit of a network where people can get together.
>
> (Injured male, KAFC)

Social ecology

This section continues with analysis of the data from the semi-structured interviews within the context of social ecology, which encompasses familial, religious and cultural resources. Within this domain there lies a pool of resources which can be utilised by individuals and communities in response to the demands and stresses experienced during complex emergencies. Figure 4.2 illustrates disrupted and reinforced resources as described by the study participants from Perth within the social ecology.

As noted, Figure 4.2 represents the disrupted and reinforced resources within the social ecology domain. The analysis revealed the categories of effects (the role played by friends), behaviour (community grief) and reactions (family emotions). The reinforced resources documented the categories of community support (bonding, making of meals, support of neighbours, spiritual support); counselling support (positive and negative reflections) and beneficial emotional support (family support). Each of these are further explained next.

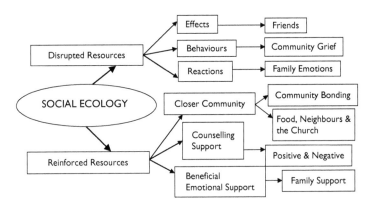

Figure 4.2 Social ecology – Perth

Disrupted resource 1: effects

Sub-theme: friends

The players who travelled to Bali had a wide circle of friends from their school days, work environments, neighbourhood and football club. On hearing the news about the dead and injured players in Bali, many young people became deeply distressed and concerned for their friends. They gathered together, near the family homes of the deceased or injured, to grieve, to wait for further news and to collectively support each other and the affected family members. This group of people are termed secondary-level victims (Alexander, 2005; Rao, 2006). They displayed reactions such as sadness, confusion and a need to be together for support. They too had become indirect victims of the attack, illustrating the terrorist aim of going beyond the direct victims of the attack to spread fear among civilians (Miller, 2004). The mother of a son killed in the bombing describes how her son's girlfriends and friends came to collectively grieve and to support her:

> She . . . [grieving girlfriend] turned up with some of . . . [deceased son's] friends that I hadn't met. She and . . . one of my son's other friends turned up and they were there from the word go and they were there for three weeks.
> (Mother of deceased male, KAFC)

Another mother described how her son's friends reacted to the news that her son had been injured and others had been killed:

> . . . [her injured son] had a very close friend who lived on the other side of Kingsley and I almost heard his car start up at about 5.30 am. He'd heard it on the news and he came screaming over. He was sitting on the front fence crying. We'd go out and three or four young men would be sitting in the car crying.
> (Mother of injured male, KAFC)

This mother describes the reaction of her son's former coach:

> One man who was a previous football coach of . . . [her injured son] and he was in his car across the road. He said 'I don't know what to say to you. Is he alright?' He couldn't get out of the car; he couldn't walk across the road.
> (Mother of injured male, KAFC)

Disrupted resource 2: behaviours

Sub-theme: community grief

While the community were extremely sympathetic to and supportive of all of the victims and family members, the Kingsley and surrounding communities also grieved for the loss of the young men from the football club. At times this made life difficult for bereaved families and appeared to compound their grief almost every time they stepped out of their house to attend to everyday tasks. Communities of Perth and Kingsley had no previous experience in dealing with victims and families of those affected by a terrorist attack, so they offered well-meaning support in the best way they could. At times participants described this as over-bearing and said it meant that the community almost took over 'ownership' of the grief and distress, as described by one mother. The following quotes by two mothers, one of a young injured male and one of a young man who was killed in the bombing, portray this sense of ownership.

> If anybody in the community realised that you were directly involved and they asked you how you were, they usually burst into tears before you did.
>
> (Mother of injured male, KAFC)

> If a car accident happened people would commiserate with you. And they move on with their lives, but Bali was owned by many Australians. It's quite a different thing, so the emotional impact was different. People just thought they owned you. It was like everybody had to share the bad for me and felt bad for themselves and felt bad for Australia with me. I'd go to the shops and someone would go oh . . . [mother's name] and put their arms around me in the middle of the shopping centre or the middle of Dewson's [local grocery store] and I found myself getting a phobia about shopping. . . we as a family had to deal with the wider community's grief.
>
> (Mother of deceased male, KAFC)

Disrupted resource 3: reactions

Sub-theme: family emotions

Family members back in Perth were also deeply affected by the events and were struggling to cope. Accurate information was initially scarce and its gathering was limited to a single player's mobile phone. As a volunteer counsellor with the football club, the researcher's (the first author) advice was constantly sought in order to provide phone support and respond to queries from family members, friends of the victims and club officials. The stress of the event seemed to take its toll on family members' psychological well-being. For a number of families the situation made for difficult relationships, which for some continued for several years. As was the case for the primary-level victims, life would not be quite the same again for the affected family members and friends.

The interviewees described the enormous shock of being informed their sons had been involved in the bombing. This was detailed in the words they were expressing as well as in the pain etched on their faces as they retold their story.

There seemed to be a mixture of initial shock and horror regarding what had happened, as well as despair and confusion surrounding how they should react to their injured, or in some cases their grieving, sons and daughters. They worried about what to say, what to do, whether their actions or words would cause more harm to their sons. There was a sense that they were 'learning on the job' and responding as they received information.

> My dad is not an emotionally dramatic guy but he was upset. Everyone in my family was so upset. . . Family-wise we were emotional, irrational and turbulent.
>
> (Injured male, KAFC)

> We were very snappy with each other. Our concentration levels suffered. You don't know how to react or respond in that situation.
>
> (Mother of injured male, KAFC)

> They were terribly shaken. My dad was just a mess.
>
> (Friend of deceased male, KAFC)

Sadly, in one family the stresses and strains continued and eventually created an emotional distance that, to date, has not been repaired. This is the case of the young man who reported that his family didn't understand why he was feeling so bad and were suggesting it was time he moved on. This has resulted in him experiencing some distance from his family. The young man reported:

> I'm not so close with my parents. I'm not saying we weren't close before but I have noticed a major distance [in 2008] among my family.
>
> (Friend of deceased male, KAFC)

Reinforced resource 1: closer community

Sub-theme: community bonding

Community members were in shock but rallied behind the young men, their families and the families of the bereaved. This stage of psychosocial care in the form of community support and consolation is part of what is termed 'psychological first aid' (National Child Traumatic Stress Network and National Center for PTSD, 2005). A prime example of how the community responded to the tragedy was the memorial service held shortly after the surviving members of the football club returned to Perth.

A number of participants described their surprise at the extent of the community support they received, and how there seemed to be a bond which they had not previously experienced. They cited the memorial ceremony as a good example of the bonding of the victims, family members and the football club.

It seemed the entire local community of Kingsley and surrounding districts turned out to celebrate the return of the injured men and offer support for the families of the missing young men. The emergency support committee that organised the memorial service presumed the number of attendees would be around 300 and were surprised when approximately 10,000 people turned up. The quotes below document the extent of the overwhelming support:

> Anyone who lived in Kingsley was affected because it was like the football club. I was directly affected but I'm sure the entire community was definitely affected.
>
> (Injured male, KAFC)

> It gave everybody something in common. . . People seemed to be communicating more. It did make the community feel closer at the time.
>
> (Injured male, KAFC)

> The big thing [the memorial ceremony week 2] at the footy club had 10,000 people turn up. . .
>
> (Injured male, KAFC)

Reinforced resource 2: community support

Sub-theme: food – neighbours and churches

The community support was intensive and varied and included food, emotional and spiritual support and information. It seemed that just as much as the shocked community members were helping the victims, the helpers also derived benefit from their actions. Supporting others affected by the tragedy appeared to help them deal with their own emotions and gave them a sense of purpose and direction at such a difficult time. Neighbours, close friends and family members undertook multiple supportive roles by shopping or cooking food for the victims, giving emotional support and acting as chauffeurs when needed.

Close friends who had grown up with the primary-level victims were a particular source of almost constant emotional support. Many stayed with the victims in their homes or made themselves available at a moment's notice to offer support. The local churches gave spiritual support in the form of prayers and also food and accommodation for those from out of town who rushed to Perth on hearing the news a family member had been injured.

The football club, its members and the committee gave much-needed emotional support and supplied crucial information to the victims regarding counselling support and financial assistance, made funeral arrangements and organised wakes via a weekly newsletter. The football clubrooms became a focal point for emergency meetings and for distressed victims, family and club members to congregate for mutual support. This enormous and continued outpouring of support for the participants is part of the community's becoming an active contributor to the recovery process and an indicator of the community's resilience (PWG, 2003).

> People I hardly knew left food on the doorstep. I didn't cook for almost three months. The local churches were very supportive too. Most of the schools in the area were affected. As each of the boys came home they had a banner up with thoughtful things on it.
>
> (Mother of deceased male, KAFC)

> It became a close little network down there [at the football clubrooms]. You could talk without having to explain and there were newsletters.
>
> (Mother of injured male, KAFC)

> The Kingsley church was very good and very subtle. The Kingsley footy club themselves were very genuine and very honest and very good. You sort of felt like you were part of a community. Random people would come up and give you a hug.
>
> (Injured male, KAFC)

Reinforced resource 3: counselling

Sub-theme: positive and negative experiences

The survivors, family members and all close relatives of the deceased were offered counselling, but there was fragmented supply and take-up of the counselling services. Services such as psychologists in private practice, psychologists from the Department of Community Development and the Red Cross were made available. In the aftermath of the bombing, and for a number of months following, the psychologists worked long and irregular hours and gave up much of their free time in an effort to intensively support the victims and their family members and friends.

The participants' experiences of counselling varied. The mothers interviewed tended to report positive experiences, while some of the injured males tended to report negative experiences of counselling. For example, an injured male described his visits to a government-provided counsellor as negative; unfortunately, the victim's perception of what happened in the counselling sessions discouraged him from attending further sessions and deprived him of the support he needed. Another described the physical and psychological reactions he experienced following his appointments with the counsellor. Regrettably, due to his own experiences, he admitted discouraging others from attending the counselling sessions.

A mother described the support group she attended at the football club, which was run by two local psychologists who volunteered their time to help the victims:

> Yes I found it helpful [the support group for family members whose sons had returned injured] because it gave me something to do. Just talking, be it about the Bali bombing, or what the kids have done at home. I just found it was something I needed to do at the time.
>
> (Mother of injured male, KAFC)

There were positive comments regarding the Red Cross, volunteer and Department of Community Development counsellors. The negative comments related to the approach of the Centrelink counsellors and the reactions displayed by government-provided counsellors:

> All of you did an amazing job in the first few weeks. We had people from the Red Cross, everybody who needed to be there was there. My Centrelink counsellor that they assigned me to in Western Australia wasn't that great, more prying than supportive. I didn't feel the person they assigned me to was adequately trained to cope with the depth of emotions.
>
> (Mother of deceased male, KAFC)

> I tried it twice. The first time [he attended] the counsellor broke down more than I did; that was a government one.
>
> (Injured male, KAFC)

It is important to note that, due to the horrific nature of the tragedy, the information revealed in the counselling sessions was very difficult for most psychologists and counsellors to hear. All were encouraged to seek peer debriefing to help them cope with the enormity of what they were hearing.

> I went there for a couple of months and every week you feel sick in your stomach when you turned up because you're back there and they look at their watch, 'Thanks a lot, we'll see you next week'. The problem is you're stuck on the last sentence for the whole week.
>
> (Injured male, KAFC)

The reality is that most government bodies that offer counselling have a waiting list and weekly sessions are often arranged as part of the overall therapeutic approach, as more than one session in a week may in some instances be counter-productive to the client's progress. As a rule most therapists advise the client that if they have a problem between sessions, telephone contact or other arrangements can be made.

I went to a group session. I really didn't get a lot out of it for me personally and then I think I went to one individual session after that.

(Injured male, KAFC)

My therapy was talking to the boys [the other victims]. That's what helped me. When I thought I needed someone to talk to, I would ring the boys [other victims].

(Injured male, KAFC)

Reinforced resource 4: most useful emotional support

Sub-theme: family support

Apart from needing medical care for their injuries, the victims were emotionally distraught and needed support due to the emotional trauma they had experienced. The following statements were made in reply to the question asking participants to detail the most useful non-medical emotional support. Initially, primary and secondary-level victims seemed to withdraw and seek support from within the immediate family unit. Eventually support also came from outside sources, such as neighbours and the wider community. This support became a reinforced link with the wider community and other extended family members.

My family, because I have got such support I think anybody that didn't have any family support or a unit out there would have been very isolated.

(Mother of injured male, KAFC)

If you've got good family support I think that makes a huge difference in the way you react to anything like that because they gathered immediately. My family support made a huge difference. My brother turned up. . . two sisters and their husbands and kids. Mum and Dad were there by 11 am in the morning.

(Mother of deceased male, KAFC)

The effect on victims' siblings was profound, and many took time off work or school to take on a supportive role within the family unit. The following mother tells a story that was repeated in many families. She described how her son and daughter became a major source of support for her, in almost a traditional role-reversal. Interestingly, this is the same family who were documented earlier in this chapter as reporting that they 'became very snappy with each other'.

You tell one and then my household was full of support. My youngest son became more supportive. My daughter went into a supportive role with me.

She took two or three weeks off her work and ran my business for me. Because I had so much support I think anybody that didn't have any family support or a unit out there would have been very isolated.

(Mother of injured male, KAFC)

Family members often helped with the practical aspects of running a household. They cooked, cleaned, did the shopping and generally looked after the victims as best they could. They also drove them to appointments in the weeks and months following the bombing, during which time there were many visits to doctors, medical specialists, psychologists and Centrelink.

Culture and values

In this section, analysis of the data from the semi-structured interviews with victims of the 2002 Bali bombings in Perth continues in the context of the domain of culture and values. According to the work of the PWG (2003), this domain encompasses human rights, cultural values, beliefs and practices, and it is these elements that are disrupted in complex emergencies. This disruption can result in an 'undermining of values, beliefs and practices' (Strang and Ager, 2005, p. 3), which is understandable, as people struggle to comprehend why such catastrophic events occur. As the victim's human rights to safety had been severely affected by the Bali bombing, in Perth many turned to the comfort of their beliefs and practices, which form the core of most societies, particularly in difficult times. The resources within this domain are illustrated in Figure 4.3.

Figure 4.3 presents disrupted resources under the category of *media interest*, which included the positive and negative aspects of the media's involvement with the tragedy and its victims. The reinforced resources were *religion*, which included the victims' return to spiritualism, and *support*, which included the mateship and

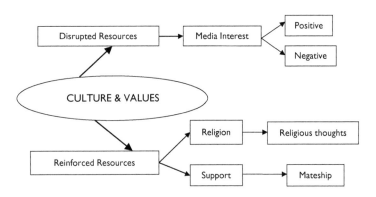

Figure 4.3 Culture and values – Perth

camaraderie that evolved among primary-level victims. These resources draw and build on the culture and values domain, and are further explained in the following sections.

Reinforced resource 1: religion

Sub-theme: religious thoughts

Most participants had attended church at some juncture in their lives. A number of participants reported returning to religious thoughts or conversations with God. Members of churches from all dominations were involved in the support of individuals and families. All recollections regarding this type of support were positive.

> I had a few conversations with God. I suppose that helps. It's a sort of love/ hate relationship we have. I felt the religious groups, regardless of their religion, were very supportive.
>
> (Mother of deceased male, KAFC)

> I didn't go back to church, but you went back to thanking God that you were the lucky one.
>
> (Mother of an injured male, KAFC)

Reinforced resource 3: support

Sub-theme: mateship

The young men in Perth spent many hours in each other's company in the days and months following the bombing. They supported each other by sharing their innermost thoughts, by their own admission drinking copious amounts of beer together and rallying to support each other when any one of the 'team' reported feeling down. They kept their mobile phones on day and night for months following the event and would often talk into the early hours of the morning. If they went out, they went out as a group, as being in a group afforded them feelings of security and safety. This was an example of what Australians call 'mateship' at its best, despite recent research which suggests this characteristic is in decline in Australian culture (Butera, 2008).

> Yes, all the guys were fantastic. If one guy is down, one guy won't get around to him, we'll all get around to him and help him out.
>
> (Injured male, KAFC)

> We stayed as a group. We were safe. We were all exactly the same way. We would not leave that little area until we went out as a group. No one went out by themselves. It went on for days, at least six or seven months.
>
> (Injured male, KAFC)

Disrupted resource 1: media interest

Sub-theme – positive and negative experiences

The local and worldwide media interest in the story was intense for days and months following the bombing. Victims, family members and friends were frequently and constantly asked for media interviews. The victims' and family members' reactions to the media interest were mixed.

> The *West Australian* was amazing; they let me write my own story. Some were real cowboys and [had] no respect for anybody. . . I just believe in a little ethical training and some respect. They need to have some kind of training so they can approach grieving people appropriately.
>
> (Bereaved mother)

> I hated the media and the way they acted. Especially when you are trying to have breakfast and they are up next to you. None of us really ate, we all tried to.
>
> (Injured male, KAFC, referring to the time in Bali)

Summary

This chapter explored analysis of the interview data from the victims in Perth. The analysis, using the lenses of disrupted and reinforced resources, has revealed that the participants' experiences are not all negative and emotionally charged. Emerging from reports of disrupted resources such as physical, psychological and emotional distress, risk-taking behaviours and community grief are stories and experiences of reinforced resources, such as churches, friends, family members, neighbours and the government, who rallied to offer practical, emotional and financial support. The information shared within this chapter has been a valuable source of information in developing the recommendations and the modified framework outlined in chapter 8.

References

Ai, A. L., Cascio, T., Santangelo, L. K., and Evans-Campbell, T. (2005). Hope, meaning, and growth following the September 11, 2001 terrorist attacks. *Journal of Interpersonal Violence, 20*(5), 523–548.

Alexander, D. A. (2005). Early mental health intervention after disasters. *Advances in Psychiatric Treatment, 11*, 12–18.

Australian Bureau of Statistics (2008). *1367.5 – Western Australian statistical indicators, June 2008: Labour market*. Retrieved 20 Aug 2014 from http://www.abs.gov.au/AUSSTATS

Australian Government (n.d.). *Overview of school education, Australia.* Retrieved 20 Aug 2014 from http://www.aei.gov.au/AEI/CEP/Australia/EducationSystem/School/Overview/default.htm

Australian Government, Australian Institute of Family Studies (2008). *Family Facts and studies. Median age at first marriage 1966–2008.* Retrieved 20 Aug 2014 from http://www.aifs.gov.au/institute/info/charts/marriage/median.html

Australian Institute of Company Directors (2007). *Western Australia: An economy on the move – Riding the boom.* Retrieved 20 Aug 2014 from http://www.companydirectors.com.au/NR/exeres/888FEB6E-7B76-475F-91F6-51A4103583A4.htm

Blanchette, I., Richards, A., Meinyk, L., and Lavda, A. (2007). Reasoning about emotional contents following shocking terrorist attacks: A tale of three cities. *Journal of Experimental Psychology, 115*(1), 47–56.

Butera, K. (2008). 'Neo-mateship' in the 21st century: Changes in the performance of Australian masculinity. *Journal of Sociology, 44*(3), 265–281. doi: 1557972201

Davis, J. L., Byrd, P., Rhudy, J. L., and Wright, D. C. (2007). Characteristics of chronic nightmares in a trauma-exposed treatment-seeking sample. *American Psychological Association, 17*(4), 187–198.

Duckworth, A. L., Steen, T. A., and Seligman, M. E. (2005). Positive psychology in clinical practice. *Annual Review of Psychology, 1,* 629–651.

Holmes, L. (2005). Marking the anniversary: Adolescents and September 11 healing process. *International Journal of Group Psychotherapy, 55*(3), 433–442.

Linley, P. A., Joseph, S., Harrington, S., and Wood, A. M. (2006). Positive psychology past present and (possible) future. *The Journal of Positive Psychology, 1*(1), 3–16.

Meisenhelder, J. B., and Marcum, J. P. (2009). Terrorism, post-traumatic stress, Coping strategies, and spiritual outcomes. *Journal of Religion and Health, 48*(1), 46–57.

Miller, L. (2004). Psychotherapeutic interventions for survivors of terrorism. *American Journal of Psychotherapy, 58*(1), 1–16.

Moore, B. (2006). Blast injuries – A pre hospital perspective. *Journal of Emergency Primary Health Care, 4*(1), 1–13.

Moore, R. S., Cunradi, C. B., and Ames, G. M. (2004). Did substance use change after September 11th? An analysis of a military cohort. *Military Medicine, 169*(10), 829–832.

National Child Traumatic Stress Network and National Center for PTSD (2005). *Psychological first aid: Field operations guide.* Retrieved 20 Aug 2014 from http://www.vdh.state.va.us/EPR/pdf/PFA9-6-05Final.pdf

Park, C. L., Aldwin, C. M., Fenster, J. R., and Snyder, L. B. (2008). Pathways to post-traumatic growth versus posttraumatic stress: Coping and emotional reactions following the September 11, 2001 terrorist attacks. *American Journal of Orthopsychiatry, 78*(3), 300–312.

Psychosocial Working Group (PWG) (2003). *Psychosocial intervention in complex emergencies: A framework for practice.* Working Paper, Centre for International Health Studies, Queen Margaret University, Edinburgh.

Rao, K. (2006). Psychosocial support in disaster-affected communities. *International Review of Psychiatry, 18*(6), 501–505. doi:1237467351.

Strang, A. B., and Ager, A. (2003). Psychosocial interventions: Some key issues facing practitioners. *Intervention, 3*(1), 2–12.

Tatar, M., and Amram, S. (2007). Israeli adolescents' coping strategies in relation to terrorist attacks. *British Journal of Guidance and Counselling, 35*(2), 163–173.

Vlahov, D., Galea, S., Ahern, J., Rudenstine, S., Resnick, H., and Kilpatrick, D. (2006). Alcohol drinking problems among New York City residents after the September 11 terrorist attacks. *Substance Use and Misuse, 41*(9), 1295–1311.

Watchorn, J. H. (2001). *Surviving Port Arthur: The role of dissociation in the impact of psychological trauma and its implications for the process of recovery.* Retrieved 20 Aug 2014 from http://eprints.utas.edu.au/1271/

West Australian Industrial Relations Commission (2007). *Minimum Wage Award.* Retrieved 20 Aug 2014 from http://www.wairc.wa.gov.au/Pages/AwardsAgreements/ AwardsAgreements.aspx

Chapter 5

Other victims: who are they?

Introduction

This chapter examines the role and contribution of volunteer responders and key informants in Bali and Perth, identified as third-level victims (TLV). The domains of human capacity, social ecology and culture and values (PWG, 2003) have again been used to underpin analysis of the interviews with volunteer responders and key informants. The initial discussion explores the roles that volunteers undertook in Bali either at ground zero very soon after the bombing occurred or in the hospital or morgue. The volunteers described working in very difficult circumstances with little or no specialised equipment, direction or training to prepare them for their roles. Trained and untrained volunteers came to help in the confusion and melee of the night. Most struggled to comprehend what had happened. The chapter commences with a brief overview of the effect on third-level victims.

Effects on third-level victims – an overview

A recognised gap in previous research led to new studies which have identified a third level of victim, such as recovery and clean-up workers (Stellman *et al*, 2008) and professional and volunteer responders (Perrin *et al*, 2007; Renholm, 2011). These third-level victims are increasingly becoming a focus of research, as it is recognised that the difficult tasks they undertake have a detrimental effect on their psychological health. Therefore a third tier of victims emerges from among the many volunteer and professional responders who work tirelessly in the aftermath of complex emergencies.

In the aftermath of a terrorist attack, many people are, as a result of their profession, required to attend the scene; these include police officers, ambulance drivers, doctors and nurses and firemen. Others, such as volunteers who were close to the scene, rush to the scene to help in the rescue effort. A plethora of studies in the area are still emerging from the 9/11 attacks, as the events of 9/11 exposed many recovery workers and volunteers to distressing scenes involving thousands of deceased victims and body parts.

The PTSD symptoms noted in these workers have been said to be comparable to those of combatants returning from the war in Afghanistan, and in some victims were still present some five years after the event (Stellman *et al*, 2008). It has also been noted that the nature of the tasks undertaken by workers seemed to influence the prevalence of PTSD symptoms. For example, workers who had to dig by hand to recover the many victims and body parts buried in the rubble of the demolished buildings demonstrated a higher level of PTSD symptoms than other on-site workers, such as the security police or rubbish removalists (Stellman *et al*, 2008). However, it must be recognised that the security personnel, police and rubbish removalists were also likely to endure a considerable amount of distress as a result of the jobs they had to undertake.

Primary and secondary-level victims, as previously discussed, often require support from mental health professionals such as psychologists, mental health nurses and social workers. The support professionals give in disaster situations is often intense and involves listening to details that are difficult for the mental health practitioner to hear. Post-disaster support is not usually a feature of their training; as a result, most rely on their professional instincts to support the victims in the best way they can. Even when post-disaster support is a feature of training or the health professional has experience in dealing with clients who have been involved in a terrorist attack, it can incur a degree of distress on a personal level. For example, in Israel, where numerous terrorist attacks have occurred, PTSD and emotional distress have been noted in social workers who treat victims (Dekel *et al*, 2007).

Similarly, social workers in New York reported secondary traumatic stress symptoms after 9/11 (Pulido, 2007). What made 9/11 support work unique is that many of the mental health professionals had been caught up in the disaster themselves, as they witnessed the attacks or lived nearby. Many reported they held their own emotions in check in order to support their clients, with a number reporting symptoms similar to those demonstrated by their clients some two or three years after the attacks (Pulido, 2007). This is similar to the effect noted in secondary-level victims who are required to intensively support their family members.

The title of third-level victim has also been given to those who live close to the scene of a disaster, or who watched traumatic scenes unfold on the television. Living close to the scene of a disaster can be enough to trigger PTSD-type symptoms, in some instances three to four times higher than in the general population (Mitka, 2008). Nearby residents in New York and Bali were exposed to the sights, sounds and smells of the disaster in the nearby streets and skyline for days after the attack. Even watching traumatic scenes on the television has been said to contribute to PTSD symptoms in some viewers (Propper *et al*, 2007), as the media (and particularly television) plays a role in disseminating the distressing scenes directly into our living rooms. It is also important to note, however, that not all the effects of terrorist attacks are deemed negative by the victims. Many report positive emotional growth after the attacks, particularly in relation to closer relationships with their family and friends and new and positive perspectives on life (Walsh, 2007), with many embracing new tasks and experiences (Bonanno *et al*, 2007).

Profile of the Bali volunteers: ground zero and hospital

Many community members and members of groups such as the Red Cross responded to help during the crisis. They worked tirelessly without regard for their own needs and sometimes safety. When reference is made to 'ground zero' in Bali, the participants are referring to the area in and around Paddy's bar and the Sari club, which were destroyed during the bombing, and where most of the dead and injured were found. Six volunteer responders were interviewed for this study:

- Two were male Red Cross members who initially worked at ground zero, and later at the morgue in Sanglah hospital.
- One female volunteer worked at Sanglah hospital in an administration role, dealing with telephone and face-to-face enquiries from relatives and friends of the victims. Another volunteer was a counsellor at the hospital, who also helped with clinical duties on the wards.
- The remaining volunteers, one male and one female, were members of the Courts organisation who helped to raise funds and distribute basic goods to the families of victims who were killed or injured in the bombing, particularly in the first few weeks following the bombing.

The volunteer reports catalogue episodes of significant psychological distress while undertaking their volunteer roles in the days, months and even years following their interventions. As in previous chapters, the analysis of their interviews commences within the context of human capacity.

Human capacity: volunteers – Bali

The following accounts describe this group of volunteers' distress and significant disruption of resources within the context of human capacity. Figure 5.1 illustrates the disrupted and reinforced resources that emerged from the analysis of the interviews with the volunteers in Bali. Effects included the emotional numbing, flashbacks, nightmares, discrimination and scapegoating that many victims experienced. Behaviour was extended to include the confusion and conflict which occurred at ground zero and in the main hospital, plus the anxiety some victims experienced in crowded places. The reinforced resources documented the categories of positive reflections – the excitement of helping, with suggestions for improved co-ordination of volunteers and the wish for fighting to stop. Each of these resources are further explained in detail below.

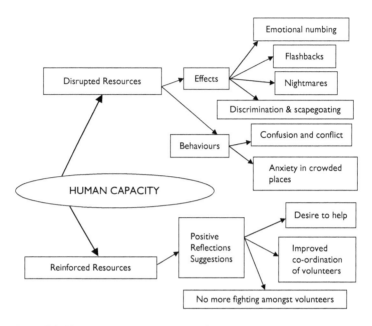

Figure 5.1 Human capacity – volunteers: Bali

Disrupted resource 1: effects

Sub-themes: emotional numbing, flashbacks, nightmares

Although they were not direct victims of the attack, the conditions in which they worked and the scenes they witnessed on the night suggest that some form of emotional first aid would have been useful support for this group of responders. In any complex emergency situation it is the victims who need to be given priority in the initial stages. However, emergency first responders can be emotionally and sometimes physically harmed by the tasks they are required to undertake. Following the second Bali bombing in 2005 and the Indian Ocean tsunami, counselling support was made available to all Red Cross volunteers.

A middle-aged female hospital volunteer felt justifiably proud at how she coped with the difficult tasks she undertook. As with most of the volunteers interviewed, this was not without personal cost, as it was 12 months before she could, as she describes, 'leave it' (her thoughts) behind. This volunteer also admitted in a statement later that some of the images she saw in the morgue are still with her, and are distressing. She described a shutting down of her emotions, 'not being able to feel anything' – a form of emotional numbing which was her emotional response to the scenes she witnessed, especially in the morgue and in the work she had to undertake. A young deceased girl she saw there reminded her of her own daughters. She said:

> I felt strong. I never imagined I could do a thing. I didn't feel anything at that time. . . It took me a year before I could leave it behind [the images]. . . I remember a young girl [in the morgue], she was beautiful. I felt sad and left after ten minutes; the images are still there.
>
> (Hospital Volunteer 1)

The Red Cross volunteers interviewed undertook a number of roles at the morgue and ground zero, in an extremely difficult environment. They assisted with body and body-part recovery at ground zero, in addition to the initial forensic examinations at the morgue. According to Hospital Volunteer 1, the morgue was hot, humid and overcrowded, with insufficient cooling, ventilation, storage space for the deceased or personal protective clothing. Stress reactions in Red Cross workers are not uncommon, as they are often the first workers to attend a disaster scene. McCaslin *et al* (2005) found that Red Cross volunteers experienced extreme stress due to prolonged exposure to the event by virtue of working long, tiring shifts which entailed dealing with bereaved relatives and survivors. The interview responses that follow give some insights into the effects at the individual level.

A Red Cross volunteer was significantly distressed following his role in the response. He said when he closed his eyes he repeatedly 'saw' the awful sights he witnessed at ground zero and in the morgue, and was afraid to close his eyes due to these flashbacks.

> For six months after the bomb I was unable to close my eyes, I had rapid hair washes. I got angry very easily. I wanted to stay alone; sometimes I cried alone.
>
> (Red Cross Volunteer 1)

These symptoms lasted for six months after the bombing. The volunteers and workers exposed at this level often become third-level victims (Alexander, 2005; Rao, 2006). Stellman *et al* (2008) reported that the levels of distress and PTSD symptoms of 9/11 volunteers were comparable to combatants returning from a war rotation in Afghanistan. The study reported significant and ongoing symptoms of flashbacks, anxiety, anger and withdrawal.

A female hospital volunteer also described having significant signs of psychological distress which lasted for some months after the bombing. She has recurrent trauma that is triggered each year at the anniversary of the bombing. The bombing also changed this volunteer's long-term overseas study plans: she decided to remain in Bali, and started up her own low-cost counselling practice.

It did change my life. I didn't go back and take that wonderful job. I didn't go on to finish my prospectus [complete her counselling thesis in America]. I think for four or five months after the bombing I had my own case of PTSD. I had a lot of nightmares a lot of difficulties. . . It's almost like there is another tragedy, someone else can deal with it because I can't handle it. Every year on the anniversary it all comes back.

(Hospital Volunteer 2)

Sub-theme: discrimination and scapegoating

The volunteers were asked to comment on the bombing's effects on the community. Communities in Bali are tight-knit, especially in the small villages, where everyone knows everyone else. Migrants from other regions of Indonesia who come to live in the villages in Bali are not easily included in village life, and it takes time to earn community trust. Even before the bombing there was mistrust and suspicion between communities, particularly between the Hindu and Muslim communities (Participant personal communication, 29 January 2002). This type of mistrust had previously been aroused in many nations following 9/11, when the 'War on Terror' campaign was launched with a 'global crusade' against 'Islamic terrorism' (Noor, 2006, p. 30). The bombing in Bali magnified this mistrust, and it was a theme highlighted in a number of volunteer and victim interviews:

If [they are] not from Bali, there is discrimination between communities.

(Red Cross Volunteer 1)

In some areas there is still [in 2008] discrimination [between the Balinese and Muslim communities], some deep emotion.

(Red Cross Volunteer 1)

Still strange, [in 2008] the community does not trust the government as much, and we suspect newcomers when they come to Bali from outside.

(Volunteer 2)

Some [of] society still feels offended with one and other [meaning between Hindu and Muslim community members].

(Red Cross Volunteer 2)

In spite of the obviously distressing effects of the bombing on volunteers, none received any formal counselling support – it was not available. One of the key recommendations from the workshop on disaster management held in Bali in 2003 was that a trauma counselling service for victims, volunteers and others be included in any future emergency plan (World Health Organization, 2003, p. 160).

Disrupted resource 2: behaviours

Sub-theme: confusion and conflict

This section details responses to the question of who took overall charge of the situation. There is often confusion in the initial stages of a disaster as many professional and volunteer personnel rush to the area to help in any way that they can. This is often a dangerous and difficult situation with little time for support and comfort, as the work needs to get done. It became clear in the interviews that the volunteering these participants undertook was not without emotional cost. Previous research has indicated that first responders, especially in disaster situations, experience intense emotional and sometimes physical responses as a result of their work (Galea *et al*, 2003).

The hospital and ground zero were overwhelmed by the number of people who responded in order to help, as well as relatives and friends of the dead, missing and injured. The situation in both venues was emotionally charged, physically demanding and difficult. There was a lack of co-ordination of volunteers at Sanglah, and this was noted at the disaster management workshop held in Bali in June 2003 (Van Bemmelen 2003; World Health Organization, 2003). The following statements detail some of the problems the volunteers experienced on the night:

> It wasn't clear who took charge. There was conflict [between volunteers].
>
> (Hospital Volunteer 1)

> It wasn't clear who took charge; there were many people: police, local rescue, Red Cross and local security.
>
> (Red Cross Volunteer 1)

Although it seems a contradictory statement, this volunteer and the one cited above explained that, while the head of the Red Cross was in charge of his members at ground zero, in the initial stages of the response no one took overall responsibility at the site:

> There was no one responsible for this. My team was headed by the head of the Red Cross.
>
> (Red Cross Volunteer 2)

Sub-theme: anxiety in crowded places

Volunteer participants reported that for a period following the bombing they were anxious when going into crowded public venues. A Red Cross volunteer describes his ongoing fear and anxiety about eating grilled food or visiting public areas because they reminded him of the sights and smells at ground zero. Yet he was able to report that not all his experiences were negative: he beamed with pride when describing how he believed he was now a 'professional' volunteer and would be able to work in any disaster situation:

> I was always afraid to go to public area[s], tourist destination[s] and shopping centre[s]. I was also afraid to eat grilled food like chicken . . . but in a positive way I was really happy to be a professional volunteer and have more motivation.
>
> (Red Cross Volunteer 2)

One of the first volunteer responders at ground zero revealed he is still fearful of crowded places. However, he can now walk around Kuta without feeling uneasy, which he was unable to do for some time after the bombing:

> Generally I can walk [around] normal already but still have . . . feelings of unease in restaurants [and] crowded places like bars and restaurants.
>
> (Volunteer Responder)

Reinforced resource 1: positive reflections/suggestions

Sub-themes: excitement of helping, improved co-ordination of volunteers, no more infighting among volunteers

Volunteers offered positive reflections on their experience during this event and suggestions to improve the experiences of volunteers responding to disasters in the future. For the following volunteer, it was less the support she received that helped her, and more having the skills and ability to help. This was a unique and isolated comment.

> My belief [that] for whatever reason that I could do something other people couldn't do at that moment. I have to say there is a bit of voyeurism of being involved, in the excitement.
>
> (Hospital Volunteer 2)

Another volunteer wanted to offer suggestions for the future in the event of a similar crisis. She had been particularly distressed by the lack of co-ordination and the infighting she observed when she worked at the hospital. She described how many people would take 'ownership' of certain tasks, such as taking telephone calls from relatives from overseas or meeting relatives, when other people had been assigned to that role. She described how women would often verbally disagree as to how best to undertake a task. The women had come together as a group from the Bali International Women's Association (BIWA). They all had particular linguistic skills and spoke a number of different European languages.

This was useful in dealing with distressed relatives from several European countries who were calling the hospital from overseas or attending the hospital in person looking for their missing relatives.

> If something like this happened again, that there be co-ordination and put [yourself] behind your organisation. Move along and do what you can – with no fighting.
>
> (Volunteer 3)

Social ecology: volunteers – Bali

Most of the emotional support for the volunteers came from family, friends and conversations with other volunteers. This form of 'non-invasive emotional support' and engagement with social networks is seen as a critical step in managing stress in volunteers (Van Ommeren *et al*, 2005, p. 73). The type of support reported by the volunteers represents the reinforced resources available in most communities, and especially in Bali, in the aftermath of a disaster. In Bali, there already existed within the community a willingness to come together and assist each other with pooling of resources (especially financial), particularly during the religious ceremonies which are culturally required after such a major incident. This pooling of resources was also very useful because of the limited support available from the Balinese government.

These support mechanisms represent a series of reinforced resources which fall under the auspice of the previously discussed domain of social ecology. This domain encompasses familial, religious and cultural resources and is illustrated in Figure 5.2. It is of note that within this domain, the volunteer participants in Bali recorded only reinforced resources.

In Figure 5.2, under the domain of social ecology, it can be seen that the interviews documented reinforced resources including positive reflections, which were expanded to include the benefits of the support of family, friends and the community, as well as recreational activities with friends and the Balinese belief system of 'letting it go'.

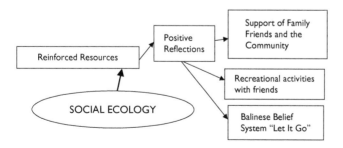

Figure 5.2 Social ecology – volunteers: Bali

Reinforced resources: positive reflections

Sub-themes: support of family, friends and the community, recreational activities, 'letting it go'

When asked about the most useful form of emotional support they received, several volunteers emphasised the importance of the support of family, friends and fellow volunteers and the benefits of being able to unwind and relax. One volunteer described his visit to the Water Bomb Park and a camping trip with friends who were not involved in the response:

> My family and friends who supported me very much. We went to Water Bomb Park [with a voucher supplied by Australian government] and camping with friends.
>
> (Red Cross Volunteer 1)

Hospital Volunteer 2, who is a counsellor in private practice, was also grateful for the support of her family and friends. Her work with clients, some of whom were involved in the tragedy, also seemed to be of benefit.

> I have family support here and friends; also the people, the clients and the patients I saw here and still see.
>
> (Hospital Volunteer 2)

A volunteer from the Red Cross sought the support of a friend who was not involved in the tragedy, as it was important for him to get away from other volunteers who wanted to continually discuss their role in the rescue efforts, which the volunteer found distressful. He described a need to get away from it all so he could try to forget.

> I talked with others involved, also a friend who wasn't involved, outside of Red Cross. I slept [at] my friend's house and he [at] mine.
>
> (Red Cross Volunteer 2)

Another hospital volunteer indicated that the support of her Balinese husband, who was also a volunteer, helped her cope, as he understood what she was feeling. She also stated her Balinese family's belief system was useful in helping her come to terms with what had happened. It taught her about accepting what had happened and letting go of painful emotions.

> The feeling of being with my husband; that helped a lot. It might have been different if he hadn't been involved. Also my Bali family, their belief system that things happen for a reason, 'this happened, so let it go'.
>
> (Hospital Volunteer 1)

Culture and values: volunteers – Bali

In Bali, religion and spiritual beliefs played an important role in the everyday lives of the volunteers. Several participants expressed that they felt the bombing had violated the spiritual balance of the island, with Muslim volunteers expressing sorrow that the actions of the bombers did not represent the religious tenets of Islam. Many participants also expressed that their religious beliefs had assisted them to cope with and recover from the effects of the bombing. These disrupted and reinforced resources are illustrated in Figure 5.3.

Disrupted resource 1: spiritual tenets

Sub-theme: disruption of spiritual values

The following participant expresses the cultural viewpoint of *Tri Hita Karana*, which is the natural balance of everyday life based on what people do, and believes the natural balance of the island had been disrupted by the bombing. He is still struggling to understand why his home, the previously peaceful island of Bali, had been a target:

> Bali is not a sacred place any more . . . I still cannot take it why Bali was the target.
>
> (Courts volunteer)

This Muslim participant was sad about the bombing, particularly as the perpetrators were believed to be Muslim. As a Muslim he believed the bombers had misinterpreted their religion, had 'got it wrong'. This viewpoint was echoed by a number of the Muslim participants and other Muslims whom the researcher encountered during her stay on the island.

> They [the bombers] got their religion wrong.
>
> (Hospital Volunteer)

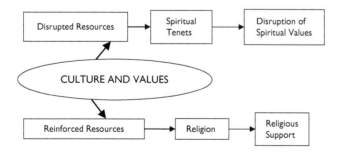

Figure 5.3 Culture and values – volunteers: Bali

Reinforced resource 2: religion

Sub-theme: religious support

As seen in the following quotes, in common with the primary and secondary-level Balinese victims, religion played an important supporting role and assisted the recovery of these volunteers:

> I am not very religious but [it was] very helpful in overcoming the problem by calling [on] God.
>
> (Hindu volunteer)

> No, I am not religious. I prayed several times with my friend and with the victims and I felt good about that.
>
> (Christian volunteer)

Key informants: Bali

Three key people from Bali were interviewed to help gain further insight into the effects of the bombing. The first informant was a Kuta village elder and local politician who arrived at ground zero very soon after the bombing and was an instrumental part of the village/community response. The second informant was a senior physician and surgeon who had operated on many of the victims through-out the night. The last informant was a senior Red Cross official who was in charge of the Red Cross response on the night.

Human capacity: key informants – Bali

Figure 5.4 is a diagrammatic representation of the themes that emerged from the key informant interview analysis in the domain of human capacity. Disrupted resources included emotional numbing of victims, fears for their children, insomnia, anxiety in the village of Kuta and burnout.

The reinforced resources revealed categories of positive reflections that included the benefits of support from peers, family friends and the community, as well as recreational activities and suggestions such as the need for specialist training and protection of Kuta.

Disrupted resource 1: effects

Sub-themes: emotional numbing – fears for children

Like other respondents who were present at ground zero and other key places, the village elder described having to suppress his sadness and fear for Bali in order to do his job. He was very proud of the way the villagers responded to the

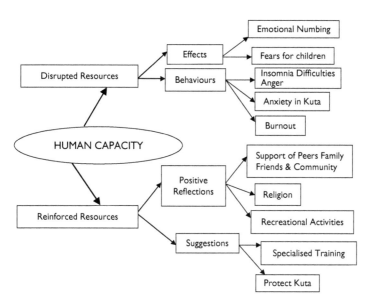

Figure 5.4 Human capacity – key informants: Bali

disaster, such as attending ground zero on the night, undertaking fire-fighting roles, rescuing the victims and donating food and rice to victims who were unable to work. As he was a leader, he felt he had to be an example to those around him and keep control. He describes having to keep his own emotions in check, similar to the Red Cross official who describes how he felt he 'had to hold onto [his emotions]'.

The elder also appeared concerned about another attack and the possibility of his children being caught up in it, and instructed his daughters to keep away from crowded places in an effort to keep them safe.

> I tried to control the emotion . . . The Kuta people were very good to the area. The villagers stood by for about one and a half months to care for the people because they were very scared. The people, the villagers, are normal. They must understand terrorists are everywhere. I tell the children [his daughters] 'Don't go to a crowded place, especially with a lot of tourists'.
>
> (Village elder)

Studies have shown that due to their involvement in a disaster, volunteers and responders often become more protective of their family members. For example, anxiety regarding their children's safety has been reported in Israeli nurses in a busy emergency-room department which deals with terrorist bomb victims on a regular basis (Riba and Reches, 2002). These effects fall under the domain of human capacity, as they have experienced a disruption to their resources – in this instance, their psychological health.

Disrupted resource 2: behaviours

Sub-themes: insomnia, anxiety in Kuta, burnout

The doctor gave an in-depth account of his role in the immediate aftermath of the bombing as the injured casualties, dead and dying came into the emergency room. The horrific scenes and treating the wounded and burnt victims were difficult experiences for the doctor and his staff. The doctor recognised his stress symptoms were serious and sought peer support. Such involvement in the treatment of so many seriously injured patients took a personal toll on him and he became very emotional when he recalled the events and his role in the response at Sanglah hospital. The researcher stopped the tape and the questioning and gave the doctor time and space to recover. Offers were made to stop or abandon the interview, which he declined.

A return to the interview occurred only when the doctor indicated he was ready to continue. The doctor recognised the toll which treating bomb victims took on the medical and nursing staff involved. He described how they worked tirelessly for days in extreme conditions for which their training had not prepared them. He also thought that some staff may be living with PTSD. His thoughts are encapsulated in his quote below:

> I couldn't believe that something like that could happen. I've never seen things like that in my life. I felt burnout and needed peer support. In terms of my profession, you have to be prepared for anything. The psychological impact to nurses, doctors and victims is ongoing. I think some of us live with post-traumatic stress disorder. I'm still deeply hurt but I try not to think about it and just work.
>
> (Senior doctor, Sanglah Hospital)

The head of Red Cross operations on the night of the bombing was responsible for co-ordinating 20 salaried staff and 71 volunteers. Here was another official who took a major role in the aftermath of the bombing, who was emotionally distressed and who also chose to carry on. In the early days he exhibited a lack of sleep and fear of loud noises, typical stress reactions to being caught up in very distressful situations. Despite his recovery from the initial symptoms the official still avoids ground zero, as it holds too many memories for him.

> I got trauma and scared with noises. I kept things in because I have a job to do [So no emotional support]. My emotions were high. I had a sleep problem [in 2002]. . . If I have a choice [in 2008] I pass by [Kuta] and do not want to go there.
>
> (Senior Red Cross official)

As in Perth, participants expressed a need to see some positive impacts from the Bali bombing, and to that end they made suggestions for strategies to assist others in any future disaster.

Reinforced resource 1: positive reflections

Sub-themes: peer, family and spiritual support; religion; recreational activities

Reflecting on and discussing the emotional support he received, the doctor referred to an informal arrangement he had with a colleague and friend. He acknowledged support and comradeship from the many doctors who volunteered their services from Australia and the Philippines and reported that casual games of ping-pong appeared to help with unwinding. Praying was also comforting for the doctor, a devout Hindu. All of the doctor's sources of support were reinforced resources already present through his friendship network, community and faith.

> I talked to a psychologist friend and I got peer support. . . Talking to friends [helped] and we faced this together and peer support. . . The support from everyone, the volunteers the medical staff from Australia and the Philippines who came to help us. . . My friends and how we helped played ping-pong. My wife and I are Hindu. It was a big help. I just prayed by myself.
>
> (Senior doctor, Sanglah Hospital)

The Red Cross official was very conscious of his role as a manager within the Red Cross. He believed his role as a leader involved the need to keep control of his emotions and avoid showing his distress to his staff. The officer reported, however, that he had received professional counselling following the Indian Ocean tsunami, when the Red Cross offered counselling to its volunteers. The official was also a deeply religious man who took a senior role in village ceremonies.

> I tried to hold onto it, I don't want to burden [anyone]. Especially as a leader I never talk. No counselling, I just kept it to myself. I try to manage it myself. I asked the God, 'Don't let it happen again'. . . Yes, it helped after the bombing. I am head of the ceremony like a priest. We have to trust.
>
> (Senior Red Cross official)

Reinforced resource 2: suggestions

Sub-themes: specialised training, protect Kuta

The doctor and the elder shared their viewpoints as to why the bombing had occurred and, in addition, the doctor made some important and useful recommendations for any future disaster response. The elder, being deeply religious, believed that everything can be managed through faith in God. He thought the bombing was a result of bad *Karma* – a reflection that the islanders had done something wrong – and felt that the bombers had tried to start a war (between the different religions) in order to destabilise Bali:

> Whatever happens they just live it and leave it to the Gods. Everything can be managed. Love to the people and love to the Gods and everything can be managed. This group was successful in bombing Bali but not successful in making Bali a war.
>
> (Village elder)

The doctor made an important suggestion regarding the need for specialised training and support of nursing and medical staff. Suggestions for change form an important part of the reinforced resources which can bring about change in any future response. The doctor was at the forefront of the response at the hospital, and recognised the psychological effects of the work on himself and other staff members.

> We need specialised training . . . For family members it was a difficult time and a big trauma and also for the doctors who try to fix the situation . . . They [the doctors and nurses] need psychological support. We need a specialised training programme and we need more medical doctors with specialised counselling training.
>
> (Senior doctor, Sanglah Hospital)

The village elder suggested there was a need to be vigilant in terms of Kuta's security:

> To keep Kuta prepared. To protect Kuta with security and support.
>
> (Village elder)

The previous sections explored the themes that emerged from the interviews with volunteers and key informants. The remainder of this chapter will be used to report on the themes that emerged from the interviews with key informants among the Perth respondents.

Key informants: Perth

The Perth key informants (KI) were all members of the Perth and Kingsley Football Club (KAFC) response team. A committee was formed at the football club to co-ordinate the response to the disaster; three of the key informants interviewed for this study were committee members. One was a politician who lived in Kingsley, the other was a media advisor in the government sector and the third was a manager of a key government department with main responsibility for co-ordinating a response to the Bali crisis. The two remaining informants interviewed were directly involved with the committee or the victims through their respective professional roles. One was a religious minister of a local church and the other a senior health professional employed in a major teaching hospital in Perth. The key topics discussed reflected those that were asked about in Bali and covered their role and training, the effects of the disaster, emotional support, coping strategies and suggestions. To preserve confidentiality, the informants have been randomly allocated the labels K1 to K5.

The response

All of the key informants were professionals – people who were most likely able to deal with difficult situations, as they sometimes occurred in their everyday occupations. However, the Bali bombing, and its effects on the football club and the local community, were not something any of the members had previously experienced. The club initially responded to the disaster without engaging outside support, until a team of local volunteers and professionals with experience in social work, psychology, media, public relations and politics quickly came together to help co-ordinate a response.

Initially, open meetings were held frequently at the football club with concerned parents and relatives of players who were seeking information and support, fearing their sons had been killed or injured. Access to valid information is a form of mutual social support and was an essential component in reducing the families' levels of anxiety and distress. It was also a useful way for the families affected by the tragedy to share their experiences and seek support from others similarly affected (Van Ommeren *et al*, 2005).

A committee of key people evolved to help with arrangements to evacuate the injured or deceased back to Perth. Other tasks involved dissemination of information by word of mouth and newsletter, investigating the legal aspects of handling a large amount of money as donations came flooding in and arranging counselling support for club members who requested it. Later the committee would be involved in arranging the memorial service for the seven dead and missing members of the club, which was attended by approximately 10,000 people from the local community. After the 13 players and members were repatriated to Perth, it was clear that many required medical treatment for their burns and other injuries. Hospital teams in Perth were put on alert immediately when the news came through of the bombing. Once casualties arrived in Perth, the medical teams worked tirelessly for many days to repair the injuries and treat the burns sustained by the victims.

Despite being busy professionals, the key informants were supportive of the study and graciously agreed to participate in the interviews. In most cases the participants were relaxed and were able to converse freely. In a few cases this appeared difficult; the researcher felt they were constrained by their professional and departmental guidelines and appeared to provide 'official' answers rather than personal responses.

Role and training

All of the key informants played an essential role in the aftermath of the bombing. Three of the five informants were connected with KAFC or lived in the locality. The fourth informant was a medical professional and the fifth a religious minister. Their particular roles meant that their contact with the injured and deceased victims' families was mainly at a professional level. At a professional level, a number of participants felt they were adequately prepared for response due to disaster protocols and training (KI 3) and training in crisis management (KI 2).

However, as one would expect, the real-life crisis was quite different to the situations that occurred in training. One participant summed this up well when he said: 'I don't know that any amount of training makes you ready for "it"'; however, another declared that training to have been 'useful'. As with the previous interviews, analysis of the Perth key informants' interviews commenced with the domain of human capacity, presented in the following section.

Human capacity – key informants: Perth

The personal and emotional toll of their roles was not initially evident to the informants. Their roles mainly involved dealing with the parents and family members of players who had been killed or injured. They were all members of the football club response committee set up to plan and organise the type of support required for the affected club members. In the initial stages, the parents and family members had no definite information about whether their sons and relatives had been injured or killed in the bombing. Most of the information was coming from the media and mobile phone calls from a few of the injured players. The toll on the committee members, who had to operate in very difficult and sensitive situations, was immeasurable, as tempers and emotions took over in the turmoil. The professional key informants, the medical professional and the local minister equally had to deal with difficult situations as they comforted or treated victims of the bombing. This is summed up particularly well by one participant:

> I think I felt like everyone else – shock at what happened. I remember going to the club, it must have been the day after because I had a feeling of the impact of war. It struck me at the time it was like a war zone; it was that sort of emotion.
>
> (KI 2)

The personal effects on key informants in 2002, and any still present in 2008, were a key focus for discussion during the interviews. Figure 5.5 illustrates the themes that emerged from these discussions within the domain of human capacity.

Figure 5.5 draws on the interviews with key informants under the domain of human capacity. The 'effects' category included emotional numbing and official versus personal responses. 'Behaviours' revealed how informants and volunteers

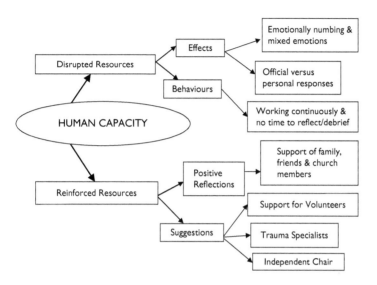

Figure 5.5 Human capacity – key informants: Perth

kept on working and had no time to reflect. Reinforced resources revealed the categories of positive reflections (the benefits to informants of support from family, friends and church members) and suggestions (the need for support for volunteers, trauma specialists and an independent chair for committees). Each of these resources are further explained next.

Disrupted resources 1: effects

Sub-themes: emotional numbing and mixed emotions

A number of informants shared, not surprisingly, that during the crisis they did not have time to process its effects. One participant reflected that 12 months after the bombing, she was emotionally drained and needed to seek emotional support as she had internalised the grief and hurt she felt. She felt she was on a treadmill and didn't realise she needed debriefing until 12 months later when her role at the football club reduced. She suggested a need for support for volunteers and committee members. This delay in processing and debriefing was reiterated by another key informant:

> . . . two weeks absolute[ly] full on, I refer to that two weeks where I actually stopped breathing. I didn't know until about 12 months later that I needed to be debriefed. I needed support.
>
> (KI 1)

I was pretty vulnerable at the time [due to personal difficulties]. You don't tend to think of things [the bombing] when you are in the thick of it. . . I didn't process it until much later. It was draining and there probably was great sadness more than anything else. It was a time of mixed emotions. I don't think anything huge, whereas I know a lot of people were hugely affected but I don't know, maybe I have become desensitised.

(KI 3)

Sub-theme: official and personal responses

Most key informants were quite sad when they discussed and reflected on the tragedy and their role in 2002, yet when asked if they were still feeling effects five years on, most appeared to deflect the question and talked instead about the effects on the victims and families. As is illustrated in the following respondent quotes, it was this question which particularly seemed to encourage what appeared to be an 'official' rather than a personal response. It may also be that this is a form of emotional numbing which helps respondents deal with the enormity of their experiences.

I almost feel a little emotional, but the overriding effect for me is my concern for the families.

(KI 2)

Five years on the effect is still with us. I don't have direct involvement with these people but you hear snippets of some people still suffering.

(KI 4)

I find it cathartic to talk about things you think about specifically. I was incredibly sad with what happened. It's something that will always be an emotional thing.

(KI 3)

Disrupted resource 2: behaviours

Sub-themes: kept on working, no time to reflect

None of the key informants received official support or counselling or, as in the case of KI 2, felt they needed it. Their responses in some ways echoed the Balinese volunteers: when in the midst of the response, primary concerns are for the victims, and any personal needs are ignored or overridden. The emotional and personal impacts appear only when their roles reduce or cease.

I internalised the grief and hurt, I didn't have an outlet. You are on a treadmill which is just going faster and faster.

(KI 1)

I don't know how it affected me in the sense I just kept going and I had the benefit of being well removed.

(KI 4)

For this participant, his extensive training and getting 'lost' in the job in hand helped him cope:

No I didn't have any counselling. I don't recall being offered any. . . You don't tend to think of things when you are in the thick of it. The training and going into surgery [helped].

(KI 3)

Reinforced resource 1: positive reflections

Sub-theme: support of family friends and church members

Despite the emotional difficulties reported, key informants discussed several positive outcomes associated with the experience of helping with the Perth response to the Bali bombings. Some suggested they didn't need emotional support, and what helped them cope was the fact they were helping others. The beneficial aspects of volunteering, particularly for self-esteem, have been noted in the literature (Steffen and Fothergill, 2009).

What helped me cope was feeling that I was doing something for someone else.

(KI 4)

As reported by other participants in this study, families, friends, church members and colleagues all provided avenues for emotional support:

Conversations and chats [with family and church members]. . . As far as encouragement you know when you are going 24/7 it is very draining, and they watch out for you and say 'Look, you need at least a couple of hours' sleep'.

(KI 5)

My family, particularly my wife, [gave support] and from certain colleagues there was support and frequent contact and discussion of some of the issues.

(KI 2)

Reinforced resource 2: suggestions

Sub-themes: support for volunteers, need for a trauma specialist and independent chair

At the conclusion of all the interviews, the participants were asked if they had any further comments to make. A number of the informants' responses are included here, as this was the point at which they appeared to relax and lose the caution that had previously appeared to be present. Key informants expressed the need for support for volunteers and committee members. This is a useful point as the professional counsellors involved, including the researcher, were working long hours within the football committee, along with their normal daytime occupations. Most volunteers were not alert to their need for support and debriefing, as the focus and priority was on the victims, the injured players and their immediate families and friends.

> One of the professionals could have made it their job to actually provide support for other volunteers.
>
> (KI 1)

The government officer made an important point in relation to the football club: he commented that it was a very tight-knit group of players and families, and it was difficult for the professionals involved to assume a directing role. He summed this up by suggesting there was a need

> to take account of the structure and work as part of it.
>
> (KI 2)

This is a very important point which ties in with Strang and Ager's research (2001, p. 6) documenting that the affected and external communities will have their own 'ecology and values'. It is important, therefore, for the external community (in this case the committee) not to try to pursue its own goals, but preferably to work within the realm of the affected community's values. In the case of the Perth victims the KAFC football community is a very tight-knit group of people with strong bonds that evolve as the players and families graduate through the various levels (junior to senior) of the club over a long period of time.

One third of the committee was known by the football club community, as they were members of the club. The remaining members, including the researcher, were not, and in some cases had no knowledge of a football community's norms and values. This resulted in the non-committee members, including the researcher, being viewed initially, and understandably, with suspicion, resulting in relationships between some club and committee members which were at times a little difficult. It took time and patience to build relationships and be accepted into the football club community. Once acceptance and trust had been built within the community, it was (and still is) like being part of a large and friendly community, whose warmth and generosity is limitless.

Another informant touched on the difficulties of having members of the affected community (the football club) sitting on the committee and being part of the decision-making process. He suggested that it would be preferable and beneficial for an outsider to chair the committee meetings:

> There wasn't one sole person, group or agency which took charge. An outside agency or person to chair the committee might have been beneficial as some

of the people on the committee were dealing with their own demons. Not that it didn't work, but it was like tiptoeing through the tulips sometimes.

(KI 2)

As in Bali, Perth participants identified problems with a lack of leadership. Many times grief and distress affected the decision-making capacity of some of the members of the committee, and this made interpersonal communications difficult, especially when tensions arose. Equally, it is not clear if the committee or football club would have responded well to outsiders taking over chairmanship of the committee. Non-members of the club were eventually accepted, as most were from the local community and/or had some form of expertise which was extremely useful in the crisis response.

A third informant also mentioned the stress within the committee and suggested an experienced trauma specialist might be useful. It is not clear if he had thought about the issue of funding for such a specialist:

It seems to me although there were people out there, the stress of the thing probably lends itself to having a top-rate trauma specialist involved.

(KI 4)

Summary

The participants offered their stories freely and willingly, as all wanted to be heard. For some it was the first opportunity to tell their story. While this study was carried out a number of years after the initial bombing, many of the participants in Bali were still reporting considerable psychological distress; however, with the help of their family members, their communities and government support all were optimistic about their future and Bali's economic survival. In Perth, the key informants all helped with the response to the disaster in Perth and reported varying degrees of distress while undertaking their professional or volunteer roles.

Both in Bali and Perth, no key informant received formal counselling support, and family, friends and colleagues seemed to be the main source of emotional support. With regard to their training the informants suggested that, in the main, their training and background were 'adequate' to help them cope with the demands of the roles they undertook in the crisis; however, most acknowledged no training could totally prepare them for the tasks they undertook. It was also acknowledged that there were difficulties involved in non-football-club members working within an already tight-knit group of people, with the result that no one person or agency with expertise took charge of the committee.

The importance of the role of third-level victims is well represented, and growing, in the literature. The current study offers a longitudinal view of the impact of terrorist attacks years after the initial event. Third-level victims provide immense support to primary and secondary victims in the immediate and longer-term aftermath of complex emergencies. Most importantly, their role is one that is part of the societal cloth through which communities move forward, and thus it is important to recognise, hear and honour their words too.

References

Alexander, D. A. (2005). Early mental health intervention after disasters. *Advances in Psychiatric Treatment, 11,* 12–18.

Bonanno, G. A., Galea, S., Bucciarelli, A., and Vlahov, D. (2007). What predicts psychological resilience after disaster? The role of demographics, resources, and life stress. *Journal of Consulting and Clinical Psychology, 75*(5), 671–682.

Dekel, R., Hantman, S., Ginzburg, K., and Solomon, Z. (2007). The cost of caring? Social workers in hospitals confront ongoing terrorism. *British Journal of Social Work, 37*(7), 1247–1262.

Galea, S., Vlahov, D., Resnick, S., Ahern, J. H., Susser, E., Gold, J. H., Bucuvalas, M., and Kilpatrick, D. (2003). Trends of probable post traumatic stress disorder in New York City after the September 11 terrorist attacks. *American Journal of Epidemiology, 158*(6), 514–524.

McCaslin, S. E., Jacobs, G. A., Meyer, D. L., Johnson-Jimenez, E., Metzler, T. J., and Marmar, C. R. (2005). How does negative change following disaster response impact distress among Red Cross responders? *Professional Psychology: Research and Practice, 36*(3), 246–253.

Mitka, M. (2008). PTSD prevalence still high for persons living near World Trade Center attacks. *JAMA, 300*(7), 779.

Noor, F. A. (2006). How Washington's 'War on Terror' became everyone's Islamophobia and the impact of September 11 on the political terrain of South and Southeast Asia. *Human Architecture, 5*(1), 29–50.

Perrin, M. A., DiGrande, L., Wheeler, K., Thorpe, L., Farfel, M., and Brackbill, R. (2007). Differences in PTSD prevalence and associated risk factors among World Trade Center disaster rescue and recovery workers. *American Journal of Psychiatry, 164*(9), 1385–1395.

Propper, R. E., Stickgold, R., Keeley, R., and Christman, S. D. (2007). Is television traumatic? Dreams, stress, and media exposure in the aftermath of September 11, 2001. *Psychological Science, 18*(4), 334–340.

Psychosocial Working Group (PWG) (2003). *Psychosocial intervention in complex emergencies: A framework for practice.* Working Paper, Centre for International Health Studies, Queen Margaret University, Edinburgh.

Pulido, M. L. (2007). In their words: Secondary traumatic stress in social workers responding to the 9/11 terrorist attacks in New York. *Social Work, 52*(3), 279–281.

Rao, K. (2006). Psychosocial support in disaster-affected communities. *International Review of Psychiatry, 18*(6), 501–505. doi:1237467351.

Renholm, D. (2011). *The psychological impact of disaster on emergency response workers, victims and communities.* Retrieved 20 Aug 2014 from http://www.slideshare.net/drenholm/the-psychological-impact-of-disaster-on-emergency-response-8371726

Riba, S., and Reches, H. (2002). When terror is routine: How Israeli nurses cope with multi-casualty terror. *Online Journal of Issues in Nursing, 7*(3), 1–5. Retrieved 20 Aug 2014 from www.nursingworld.org/MainMenuCategories/ANAMarketplace/ANAPeriodicals/OJIN/TableofContents/Volume72002/No3Sept2002/IsraeliNursesandTerror.aspx

Steffen, S. L., and Fothergill, A. (2009). 9/11 Volunteerism: A pathway to personal healing and community engagement. *The Social Science Journal, 46*(1), 29–46.

Stellman, J. M., Smith, R. P., Katz, C. L., Sharma, V., Charney, D. S., and Herbert, R. (2008). Enduring mental health morbidity and social function impairment in World Trade Center rescue, recovery, and cleanup workers: The psychological dimension of an environmental health disaster. *Environmental Health Perspectives, 116*(9), 1248–1253.

Strang, A. B., and Ager, A. (2001). *Building a conceptual framework for psychosocial intervention in complex emergencies: Reporting on the work of the Psychosocial Working Group*, 1–6. Centre for International Health Studies, Queen Margaret University, Edinburgh.

Van Bemmelen, S. (2003). Volunteer assistance at Sanglah Hospital after the Kuta blast (12-10-2002): Recommendations. In World Health Organization (Author), *Workshop on disaster management for the health sector in Indonesia, Lessons learned from the Bali Bomb* (pp. 1–18). Bali, Indonesia: WHO.

Van Ommeren, M., Saxena, S., and Saraceno, B. (2005). Mental and social health during and after acute emergencies: Emerging consensus. *Bulletin of the World Health Organization, 83*(1), 71–76.

Walsh, F. (2007). Traumatic loss and major disasters: Strengthening family and community resilience. *Family Process, 46*(2), 207–227.

World Health Organization (2003). *Workshop on disaster management for the health sector in Indonesia: Lessons learned from the Bali bomb.* Bali, Indonesia: WHO.

Chapter 6

The aftermath of terrorist attacks, including the effects and support interventions

Introduction

While recognising the difficulties individual victims experience as a result of a terrorist attack, research is now moving away from a focus on the negative effects at the individual level to studies which include an examination of the effects on the many others affected by such events, such as family members and friends (Buesnel, 2004; Stellman *et al*, 2008). There is also a proliferation of research which examines the post-traumatic growth (PTG) that many victims report following a traumatic event (Park and Helgeson, 2006). Through studies which focus on the terrorists and the attacks they undertake, evidence-based research has uncovered effective support and treatment protocols, as well as the efficacy of using a psychosocial approach in the aftermath.

The effects of terrorist acts

Increasingly, studies view the effects of terrorist attacks and disasters as multi-layered, and the effects not limited to simply physical or psychological aspects alone. For example, it is not uncommon for individual victims to report effects such as insomnia, nightmares, suppressed emotions, overuse of drugs and alcohol and intense feelings of anger (Meisenhelder and Marcum, 2009). It was noted that following the 9/11 attacks, people were found to be self-medicating as a way of relaxing or being able to cope (DiMaggio *et al*, 2009), in an effort to try and deal with the enormity of what had happened.

There is a range of psychological sequelae that emerge after such events, as inevitably all of those affected typically alter their behaviour in some way. A small proportion of the population affected by a disaster will develop post-traumatic stress disorder, and possibly specific psychiatric disorders. It is not the intent to include an in-depth discussion of post-traumatic stress and other psychiatric disorders in this section, as these are covered extensively in other publications (e.g. Neria *et al*, 2009) and they are not germane to the research study carried out in Bali. Therefore this first section includes a discussion of the concepts of post-traumatic growth and resilience and in the second section presents an overview of some of the interventions that support victims of terrorist acts.

Post-traumatic growth

Most victims exposed to a disaster or other extremely traumatic event will exhibit some signs of acute stress (Pooley *et al*, 2012). The effects of human-made and natural disasters are felt widely, from the individual directly involved to their families and the wider community. Victims may experience physical injury, psychological distress and increased alcohol and drug use (Hasin *et al*, 2007; Ford *et al*, 2006). In addition to acute stress, there are a number of studies which document that some victims detail positive effects from exposure to a disaster. Park and Helgeson report that in the aftermath of a crisis and its impacts, victims will often re-evaluate what is important to them, changing jobs, growing closer to family members and exploring new opportunities and possibilities. This phenomenon is termed post-traumatic growth (PTG) (Tedeschi and Calhoun, 2004).

PTG has been a growing area of research over the past decade and a half and there are a number of studies which now question its validity as a construct. The Canberra Bush Fire Study (Camilleri *et al*, 2007) was a study of 500 survey respondents and 40 interview participants. This study demonstrated a diversity of responses, with some participants reporting more positive ratings after the disaster (family relationships, overall level of support and spiritual beliefs) and some negative effects (friendships, work situations, financial situations and overall health) which felt worse after the disaster. This would suggest that victims may experience growth in some areas and deterioration in others (Camilleri *et al*, 2007).

Many of the studies that report PTG use self-reported questionnaires. The efficacy of their use and the construct of stress-related growth were both studied by Weinrib *et al* (2006), in whose research 163 female participants were studied for stress-related growth. In the analysis of PTG and the co-variates of severity of event and time since the event, it was discovered that women who experienced more severe events also reported more PTG on the PTG inventory. The findings supported the notion of PTG as a construct and its assessment via a self-report questionnaire.

Interestingly, other studies question the validity of individual self-reports of post-traumatic growth (Hobfoll *et al*, 2007). There is a suggestion that participants in studies of PTG which use self-report questionnaires deliberately inflate their growth experience in an effort to cope with the terrible events they have experienced (Park and Helgeson, 2006). Other studies suggest it is a cognitive distortion which occurs as victims' recollections of the past are 'derogating rather than an improvement from past to present, and is illusory' (McFarland and Alvaro, 2000, p. 340). It is likely that PTG has many facets and will vary depending on the level of the victim's distress and the magnitude of the disaster. It may be that it is a coping mechanism used during the stressful events and afterwards, or it may occur as victims realise they have actually coped with the event (Zoellner *et al*, 2008).

Resilience

Resilience is a term used frequently in research and in the popular media, and is defined in a number of ways within the literature. One such definition is that of Atkinson, Martin, and Rankin (2009, p. 137): 'the ability to return to the original form and to recover readily from the extremes of trauma, deprivation threat or stress'. Others, such as Paton, Smith, and Violanti (2000), see it as an opportunity, despite the stress, for growth to occur. Similarly, Rutter (2007, p. 208) suggests resilience is a phenomenon observed when individuals have 'relatively good outcomes despite exposure to adverse life experiences'. It has also been described by Bonnano and Gupta as 'the capacity to experience a traumatic exposure without developing PTSD' (Bonnano and Gupta, 2013, p. 146).

What binds these definitions together is that they suggest there is an element of individual recovery from difficult events. Others agree with Rutter but add that stoicism alone is not sufficient evidence, and suggest that 'positive growth' following an adverse event must be present as well (Atkinson *et al*, 2009, p. 139). Examples of resilience and growth were witnessed many times in the responses to the events of 9/11 and the 1995 Oklahoma bombing. Post-9/11, volunteers came forward in their thousands to help, numerous remembrance ceremonies were organised, volunteers helped to clean up neighbourhoods and many self-help support and advocacy groups sprang up (Walsh, 2007). It was an excellent example of communities working together with 'learned resourcefulness rather than helplessness' (Walsh, 2007, p. 222). The Bali bombing was no exception, with many volunteers willing to work in difficult circumstances at ground zero and the hospital. The irony is that the very nature of terrorist attacks is often the catalyst to motivate people to help each other.

Bonanno *et al* (2007) widen the debate surrounding an explanation of resilience to include what they believe are protective factors that may promote resilience at the individual level, such as steady income level, good social supports and a lack of chronic disease. This leads to an interesting area, where research and interventions may now be targeted to identify those most at risk due to these socio-contextual factors and can be aimed at promoting resilience and capacity-building within individuals and communities (Bonanno *et al*, 2007). The work of the Psychosocial Working Group (PWG) suggests that resilience is the extent to which communities demonstrate their ability to 'draw on their own resources' and 'meet their own needs' following complex emergencies such as terrorist attacks (PWG, 2003, p. 2).

Norris's study examined the notion that resilience was best understood and measured as just one of a set of 'trajectories' (Norris *et al*, 2009, p. 2191). The data from two studies in a four-wave longitudinal design following the floods in

Mexico in 1999[1] and the 9/11 terrorist attacks in New York were examined. The studies included 1,267 participants from New York and 561 from Mexico. Despite the difficult experiences of 9/11, the participants from New York were observed to demonstrate signs of moderate distress, which over time declined to mild and, eventually, no distress.

In Mexico, the prevalence of resilience was substantial, with participants initially demonstrating severe distress, which improved rapidly to moderate distress. From this juncture it was reported that it took a few months for this group of participants to 'bounce back' and show only mild distress. In both samples, participants also demonstrated signs of resistance (no symptoms or mild and stable), recovery (initially moderate to severe symptoms followed by a gradual decrease) and chronic dysfunction (moderate or severe and stable symptoms). It was also noted that neither set of participants demonstrated a relapsing/remitting trajectory, with New York participants being the only victims to display a delayed dysfunction trajectory.

This study demonstrated that resilience is not the only path of recovery in victims during the aftermath of a disaster. Resistance, recovery and delayed dysfunction are all possible trajectories. This information is worthy of further study as ultimately it may lead to a wider understanding of victims in the aftermath of a disaster, and 'may be of benefit to intervention programmes that aim to increase resilience and decrease adverse trajectories' (Norris *et al*, 2009, p. 2191).

In the disaster literature there are few studies exploring resilience in differing cultures, despite the suggestion that there are variations between cultures (Rajkumar *et al*, 2008), and thus resilience appears to be greatly influenced by cultural norms and values (Romero, 2011). In their study of a fishing community in Tamil Nadu, India in the aftermath of the Indian Ocean tsunami, Rajkumar *et al* (2008, p. 851) found participants demonstrated many individual coping strategies, which included 'an individual fatalistic attitude, a collective community approach to their sorrow, plus the adoption of social and spiritual barricades against the ensuing chaos and despair'.

The villagers in Tamil Nadu appeared to demonstrate what we already know from the literature: that strong connectedness with others and being able to seek reassurance and safety are all factors that can help increase resilience (Walsh, 2007). This strong community response and the need for social and cultural cohesiveness are all factors observed within the community and participants in the present study (Brookes, 2010). These are all very important factors for consideration by outside support agencies and health professionals, particularly when responding to a disaster in a non-western setting.

Collective resilience

As discussed in earlier chapters, people who have not previously met will often bond, work and stay together during high-magnitude stressful events such as terrorist attacks or natural disasters. They gather together in an effort to support each other, accept and give help such as first aid, move people to a place of safety and encourage each other throughout the event. This occurs even when there is a perceived possibility of further attacks or threats to the self, especially during natural disasters.

In this instance studies have described the phenomenon as 'collective resilience' (Drury *et al*, 2009, p. 85), as crowds or groups of people adapt to difficult circumstances and become a 'psychosocial resource'. This is in contrast to the notion often suggested in the media that there is widespread panic among victims. An excellent example of collective resilience and supportive behaviour by many people was demonstrated on the upper and lower floors of the North and South Towers of the World Trade Center attacked on 9/11. In this instance people were in the main polite and orderly and moved down the stairs in an ordered evacuation (Drury and Reicher, 2010). This lack of panic and orderly evacuation helped save many lives, as people laughed, joked and helped each other on the way down to safety, in some cases some 84 floors below (Brooks, 2005).

Interventions that help

Recognising the value of using a psychosocial approach in disaster mitigation, the Red Cross established a psychosocial support centre in 1993 (Hanson, 2009). The Red Cross also incorporated the approach into their training packages for emergency personnel (Hanson, 2009) and contributed to a joint agency framework of education and training materials aimed at community and health professionals in all states of Australia who may become involved in a disaster response (Australian Red Cross, 2009, 2013). The PWG has also produced a number of papers which contribute to the application of psychosocial work in various settings, such as East Timor (Loughry and Kostelny, 2002), Afghanistan (Loughry *et al*, 2005) and Mozambique (Boothby *et al*, 2006). It is this framework developed by the PWG that underpins the analysis of the data gathered in the Bali study. A discussion regarding a psychosocial approach to disaster support and approaches follows.

Interventions using a psychosocial approach to support victims

The psychosocial aspects of any form of disaster are numerous and go beyond the terrible tally of deaths, injuries and damage to the infrastructure of a community. Increased rates of depression, anxiety, substance abuse, risky sexual behaviour, child abuse, rape and family violence are all potential underlying effects which can occur within a family unit following any mass trauma event (Landau *et al*, 2008). For an intervention programme to be effective, it is important that support strategies are tailored to meet the specific needs of the population, otherwise gaps in support or the wrong type of support can be offered. The PWG framework for interventions is one approach which, if applied, ensures that the needs of an affected population can be comprehensively assessed and an appropriate response framework produced.

The PWG recognises the need to adopt a wide approach to explain the term 'psychosocial well-being' (PWB) and suggests it encompasses the 'social, cultural and psychological influences on well-being' (PWG, 2003, p. 1). The PWG makes several useful suggestions which aim to promote interaction and dialogue between the affected community and the external support agency (Strang and Ager, 2001). In particular, it emphasises the need to ensure that the family and community are 'brought into the picture' when assessing needs and responses. They postulate that the PWB of an individual is influenced by several key factors and stress the importance of viewing the PWB as part of a wider 'social unit', to include families, households and communities.

The three key factors or domains considered important within the framework are human capacity, social ecology and culture and values. These three key areas are interrelated, and therefore changes such as disaster effects in one area will have a detrimental knock-on effect to another area, and ultimately to the overall well-being of the people. Clearly individuals and communities do not exist independently and in complex emergencies (according to the PWG) become active contributors to their own recovery, with skills, abilities and pre-existing support mechanisms which they can tap into. The degree of this active response can be viewed as an indicator of a community's resilience (PWG, 2003).

For an intervention programme to be effective post-disaster, the PWG suggests it must aim to build the capacity of a community through an effective appraisal process. Such a programme should take into account these pre-existing resources (PWG, 2003) and occur within a process where the external support community 'collaborates and negotiates' with the affected community, particularly in a developing country. Without this process, the PWG suggests, interventions will be 'inappropriate and fail' (p. 2). As Saul and Bava (2002, p. 5) state, 'collective trauma requires a collective response'. It is therefore crucial that any evidence-based interventions and support programmes should aim to empower the victims rather than dictate to them and aim to extend the support systems that naturally occur in most communities. By helping victims tap into an easily accessible store of pre-existing resources through reconnecting with their family, their communities and their culture, the support programme will help to promote resilience in the victims and the affected community.

Research in countries such as India and Sri Lanka following the Indian Ocean tsunami supports the view that most of the victims' symptoms in the initial post-event period will abate, but this is dependent on them receiving effective social support from their family, friends and community. Social support is particularly important, as in the aftermath of any type of disaster most survivors will 'feel lonely, isolated and afraid' (Rao, 2006, p. 505), and will need to feel the comfort, support and reassurance of others (MacGeorge *et al*, 2004; Vijaykumar *et al*, 2006; Walsh, 2007).

In Japan, the psychosocial framework of response was extremely helpful as, following the tsunami and the subsequent Fukushima nuclear disaster, there was a large mobilisation of mental health workers, but it was difficult to reach all the victims – especially in the many rural areas affected. In the post-disaster analysis it was recognised that the large influx of mental health workers on the ground was not sustainable in the long term and that there was a need to strengthen the capacity of existing services. It was decided there was a need to train local community health workers. These workers would have local knowledge of the people and the area and would be aware and build on the traditional coping mechanism of Japanese people, which is not to express grief or anger, but rather to offer gentle support and move on to re-establish their communities (Yamazaki *et al*, 2011). Therefore there is a strong case for the promotion of very careful assessment, negotiation and collaboration with the local community to ensure the support fits the needs and wants of the community, and that it is distributed fairly and is sustainable.

In recognition of the overall effectiveness of a psychosocial approach, the World Health Organization produced a framework for mental health and psychosocial assistance in tsunami-affected areas (WHO, 2005). Most empirically based interventions and informed response agencies now advocate for a psychosocial approach to help meet the needs of victims. The LINC, ARISE (Landau *et al*, 2008), Psychological First Aid (Vernberg *et al*, 2008), HEARTS (Hanscom, 2001) and Hobfoll *et al*'s (2007) study have all been informed by the literature and moved away from the Critical Incident Stress Debriefing techniques once previously favoured. Central to the psychosocial approach is the desire to empower victims, provision of a place of safety and comfort, provision of practical assistance, stabilisation of their distress and promotion of connectedness and linkage with their family and their communities as early as possible.

The LINC (Linking Human Systems) community resilience model

Often the psychological effects of a disaster are a prime consideration in a psychosocial response. However, Landau *et al* (2008) highlight additional benefits not often considered in the literature, in that reconnecting victims can help mediate against the health dangers which can be triggered by mass disasters, such as heart attacks, depression and cardiac arrhythmias. Central to the LINC Model for individuals, families and communities is a response which supports and encourages individuals and families to regain self-sufficiency, rather than remain dependent on social or governmental resources. The LINC approach is cost-effective, primarily as it involves the recruitment and coaching of an individual or subset of community members who act as 'natural agents for change' (Landau *et al*, 2008, p. 197).

These family or community members become a useful link between professionals and victims, particularly in developing countries where interventions by perceived outsiders might not be culturally or socially acceptable, based on the premise that communities have historical and cultural knowledge that will also help build group resilience. The nature of the professional's involvement is purely to meet with the family link member and to offer them training, advice and support (Landau *et al*, 2008).

Psychological first aid

PFA is an approach to help reduce the stressful emotions that occur as a response to being involved in a disaster situation, such as confusion, fear, helplessness, anxiety and anger (National Child Traumatic Stress Network and National Center for PTSD, 2005). Hobfoll *et al* (2007) examined five intervention principles to guide support strategies in the initial and mid-term stages of a post-disaster response at the individual and community levels. According to the authors, the approaches have empirical support and are based on an extensive review of the literature and the extensive experience of the panel of experts brought together to produce them. The principles are to promote a sense of safety, calm, self and collective efficacy, connectedness and hope. The authors promote the need for pilot-testing of the suggestions and for their utilisation in strategic planning for future disaster response. They also caution that there is a need to avoid overstating the efficacy of interventions based on these strategies without clinical trials and further analysis. They quite rightly suggest it is likely there will not be a one-size-fits-all strategy due to the complexities inherent to all disaster situations (Hobfoll *et al*, 2007).

The PFA approach consists of eight strategies designed for use in the immediate aftermath of a disaster. They are:

- contact and engagement;
- safety and comfort;
- stabilisation;
- information gathering;
- practical assistance;
- connection with social supports;
- information on coping support;
- linkage with collaborative settings.

The Australian Red Cross promotes PFA as an approach to use in the initial post-disaster stages and beyond. The Australian Red Cross produced a comprehensive and clear booklet, *Psychological First Aid* (2013), which sets out what psychological first aid is and what it isn't, plus offering guidelines for its use. The guidelines closely reflect the eight strategies outlined above, with the ultimate aim of listening to what people want and helping them to access the basic services they may require, as well as linking them as quickly as possible with their loved ones and support networks (Australian Red Cross, 2013). The guide was produced in line with resources outlined in the Psychosocial Support in Disasters Portal (www.psid.org.au) and in the World Health Organization, War Trauma Foundation and World Vision International's *Psychological First Aid: Guide for Field Workers* (2011). All three are resources which promote gentle support and practical help for victims post-crisis and encourage support which respects the victims' 'dignity, culture and abilities'.

ARISE (A Relational Sequence of Engagement)

An extension of the LINC approach described is ARISE, 'A Relational Intervention Sequence of Engagement', which was proposed by Landau *et al* (2008, p. 200). The ARISE approach extends to families who have a member engaged in self-destructive or addictive behaviour, which can potentially occur in young victims following a disaster, as they struggle to cope with what has happened. The behaviours can be part of a pre-existing condition which is exacerbated by their experiences or a new behaviour. Again, in this treatment protocol, family members are deemed an important part of the support team. Family members are recruited, trained and supported by professionals from the ARISE team and support the family member in need by utilising natural systems of support within the family unit or extended family system (Landau *et al*, 2008). These qualitative studies demonstrate the family unit as a useful resource for professionals to utilise when responding to a mass trauma situation, particularly in a developing country.

Critical Incident Stress Debriefing (CISD)

Given that most people exposed to terrorist attacks who display symptoms of distress will eventually recover and not require clinical interventions (Mansdorf, 2008; Rajkumar *et al*, 2008), the efficacy of using CISD as an intervention technique has come to be disputed (Phillips, 2009; Sumathipala and Siribaddana 2005). CISD was based on the notion that there was a need to offer psychological debriefing to all victims exposed to a disaster. A recent review of disaster recovery literature by Winkworth (2007) documented several studies which argued CISD is an ineffective technique that can actually have an adverse effect on some victims. Instead, strategy-based models such as those described above help 'normalise' distressful symptoms as an 'understandable reaction to an abnormal event' and encourage reconnection to family and social networks (Philips, 2009, p. 86). Yet supporters of CISD suggest that critics of the approach have misunderstood the model and appraisals have taken place with inaccurate examples of the approach (Everly and Mitchell, n.d.).

HEARTS treatment model: History, Emotions, Asking, Reason and Teaching

Hanscom (2001) suggested a treatment model for victims exposed to terrorist attacks which he termed 'HEARTS', The treatment model was based on his experiences working with adults exposed to torture. HEARTS is an acronym:

- **H** is for listening to the **H**istory among others, a gentle supportive environment and listening compassionately;
- **E** is for focusing on **E**motions and reactions. This involves using good techniques such as reflective listening, asking gentle questions and naming the emotions;
- **A** is for **A**sking about symptoms, with the therapist using his or her own style to investigate current levels of physical and psychological symptoms and suicidality;
- **R** is for explaining the **R**eason for the symptoms. This means explaining the body's reactions to trauma and an emphasis on 'normal reactions and symptoms to a very abnormal event';
- **T** is for **T**eaching relaxation and coping skills such as abdominal breathing and meditation.

Overall, most contemporary approaches to post-disaster support advocate for a holistic approach which involves family members, professionals and the community in a collaborative approach which has moved away from the medical model of preferred interventions. Particularly in the initial stages of support, there will be many victims who will need some basic form of support. Because of the high numbers of victims in mass trauma situations this also makes good practical sense, as demands may quickly outstrip what the individual therapists are able to offer – hence the need for community members or 'gatekeepers such as mayors, military commanders, school teachers and lay members of the community' to be involved in the response (Hobfoll *et al*, 2007, p. 301). This argument informs a number of the recommendations listed in chapter 8 of this study. Although there are differences in some of the approaches discussed, what binds them together is the focus on an advanced emphatic alliance and empowerment of the victims.

To accompany the psychosocial approach discussed, therapists in trauma recovery now generally move away from a pathology focus (where it is assumed individuals post-disaster are likely to present with PTSD) to one in which the professional utilises approaches which promote the capacity for 'healing and resilience' that most people have (Walsh, 2007, p. 208). To assist this process it is useful if the therapist undertakes an approach which fosters 'compassionate witnessing' (Weingarten, 2006, p. 16). Compassionate witnessing requires the therapist to promote a gentle and supportive therapeutic alliance where the therapist acknowledges the loss and pain the victim has experienced, but also supports and recognises the victim's strengths and support mechanisms which are available to them within their family and communities. It is a collaborative, respectful approach which if used in the early stages following a traumatic event will reduce the likelihood of developing PTSD symptoms (Foa *et al*, 2005).

Summary

This review adds to the discussion surrounding the effects of disasters, either human-made or natural, and the support mechanisms available. It has highlighted gaps in the research and opposing viewpoints which have implications for future research. Contemporary disaster research findings are highlighted, in particular those that take a holistic and psychosocial approach to disaster mitigation. In a move away from the medical approach to trauma, a psychosocial approach is recommended which provides a way forward to help meet the multiplicity of victims' needs. It is recognised that interventions may not be required for all of the people caught up in terrorist attacks or natural disasters. In fact, many victims do not take up the offer of post-attack professional support and, in the main, do not demonstrate any increase in pathology (Mansdorf, 2008). The instinctive nature of people is to cope with extreme duress, and their resilience has generally been underestimated (Carballo *et al*, 2006, p. 223). What is required, especially in the first few days and weeks after any disaster, is the provision of safety, food and contact with others, especially family. Practical assistance and information needs to be delivered by people who are preferably local and trained in psychosocial responses which take into account local beliefs, cultural norms and practices.

Note

1   These floods, the worst for over 50 years, lasted for approximately two weeks and spread over several states in Mexico, leaving over 300,000 homeless and approximately 425 dead.

References

Atkinson, P. A., Martin, C. R., and Rankin, J. (2009). Resilience revisited. *Journal of Psychiatric and Mental Health Nursing, 16*(2), 137–145.

Australian Red Cross (2013). *Psychological first aid: An Australian guide to supporting people affected by a disaster.* Retrieved 20 Aug 2014 from http://www.redcross.org.au/files/Psychological_First_Aid_An_Australian_Guide.pdf

Australian Red Cross, Australian Psychological Society, Australian Society for Post Traumatic Mental Health (2009). *Psychosocial Support in Disasters.* Retrieved 20 Aug 2014 from http://www.psid.org.au/response

Bonanno, G. A., Galea, S., Bucciarelli, A., and Vlahov, D. (2007). What predicts psychological resilience after disaster? The role of demographics, resources, and life stress. *Journal of Consulting and Clinical Psychology, 75*(5), 671–682.

Bonanno, G. A., and Gupta, S. (2013). Resilience after disaster. In Y. Neria, S. Galea, and F. H. H. Norris (Eds), *Mental Health and Disasters* (pp. 145–160). New York: Cambridge University Press.

Boothby, N., Crawford, J., and Halperin, J. (2006). Child soldier life outcome study: Lessons learned in rehabilitation and reintegration efforts. *Global Public Health, 1*(1), 87–107. doi:10.1080/17441690500324347

Brooks, J. (2005). *Stories of September 11*. Retrieved 20 Aug 2014 from http://old. 911digitalarchive.org/stories/details/11271

Brookes, G. (2010). *The multilayered effects and support received by victims of the Bali bombings: A cross-cultural study in Indonesia and Australia*. (Doctor of Philosophy Thesis, Curtin University of Technology, Perth, Western Australia.)

Buesnel, G. (2004, 24 November). *All soldiers have nightmares*. Paper presented at the Australian Institute of Criminology Conference of Crime in Australia: International Connections. Retrieved 20 Aug 2014 from http://www.aic.gov.au/events

Camilleri, P., Healy, C., McDonald, E., Nicholls, S., Winkworth, G., and Woodward, M. (2007). *Recovering from the Canberra bushfire: A work in progress*. Report for Emergency Management Australia. Retrieved 20 Aug 2014 from http://www.dhcs.act. gov.au/data/assets/pdf_file/0009/11052/Recovering_from_the_2003_Canberra_ bushfire.pdf

Carballo, M., Heal, B., and Horbaty, G. (2006). Impact of the tsunami on psychosocial health and well being. *International Review of Psychiatry, 18*(3), 217–223.

DiMaggio, C., Galea, S., and Li, G. (2009). Substance use and misuse in the aftermath of terrorism. A Bayesian meta-analysis. *Addiction, 104,* 894–904. Retrieved 20 Aug 2014 from http://hdl.handle.net/2027.42/.

Drury, J., and Reicher, S. (2010). Crowd control: How we avoid mass panic. *Scientific American Mind,* November/December 2010, 58–65.

Drury, J., Cocking, C., and Reicher, S. (2009). The nature of collective resilience: Survivor reactions to the 2005 London bombings. *International Journal of Mass Emergencies and Disasters, 27*(1), 66–95. Retrieved 20 Aug 2014 from http://www.sussex.ac.uk/ affiliates/panic/IJMED%20Drury%20et%20al.%202009.pdf

Everly, G. E., and Mitchell, J. T. (n.d.). *A primer on critical incident stress management (CISM)*. The International Critical Incident Stress Foundation. Retrieved 20 Aug 2014 from http://www.icisf.org/inew_era.htm

Foa, E. B., Cahill, S. P., Boscarino, J. A., Hobfoll, S. E., Lahad, M., McNally, R. J., and Solomon, Z. (2005). Social, psychological, and psychiatric interventions following terrorist attacks: Recommendations for practice and research. *Neuropsychopharmacology, 30,* 1806–1817.

Ford, J. D., Adams, M. L., and Dailey, W. F. (2006). Factors associated with receiving help and risk factors for disaster related distress among Connecticut adults 5–11 months after the September 11th terrorist incidents. *Social Psychiatry and Epidemiology, 41,* 261–270.

Hanscom, K. L. (2001). *Treating survivors of war trauma and torture*. Retrieved 20 Aug 2014 from http://www.astt.org/KHanscom-article.html

Hanson, P. (2009). *Psychosocial interventions: A handbook*. International Federation of Red Cross and Red Crescent Societies Reference Centre for Psychosocial Support.

Hasin, D. S., Keyes, K. M., Hatzenbuehler, M. L., Aharonovich, E. A., and Alderson, D. (2007). Alcohol consumption and posttraumatic stress after exposure to terrorism:

Effects of proximity, loss, and psychiatric history. *American Journal of Public Health*, *97*(12), 2268–2274.

Hobfoll, S. E., Watson, P., Bell, C. C., Bryant, R. A., Brymer, M. J., Friedman, M. J., and Ursano, R. J. (2007). Five essential elements of immediate and mid-term trauma intervention: Empirical evidence. *Psychiatry, 70*(4), 283–304.

Landau, J., Mittal, M., and Wieling, E. (2008). Linking human systems: Strengthening individuals, families, and communities in the wake of mass trauma. *Journal of Marital and Family Therapy, 34*(2), 193–205.

Loughry, M., and Kostelny, K. (2002). *Mapping psychosocial interventions in East Timor.* Retrieved 20 Aug 2014 from http://www.forcedmigration.org/psychosocial/papers/PWGpapers.htm/East%20Timor%20report%20pdf.pdf

Loughry, M., MacMullin, C., Eyber, C., Abebe, B., Ager, A., Kostelny, K., and Wessells, M. (2005). *Assessing Afghan children's psychosocial well-being: A multi-modal study of intervention outcomes.* Retrieved 20 Aug 2014 from http://www.forcedmigration.org/psychosocial/pape/afghan_report_ccf_ox_qmuc.pdf

Mansdorf, I. J. (2008). Psychological intervention following terrorist attacks. *British Medical Bulletin, 88*(1), 7–22.

McFarland, C., and Alvaro, C. (2000). The impact of motivation on temporal comparisons: Coping with traumatic events by perceiving personal growth. *Journal of Personality and Social Psychology, 7*(9), 327–343.

MacGeorge, E. L., Samter, W., Feng, B., Gillihan, S. J., and Graves, A. R. (2004). Stress, social support, and health among college students after September 11, 2001. *Journal of College Student Development, 45*(6), 655–668.

Meisenhelder, J. B., and Marcum, J. P. (2009). Terrorism, post-traumatic stress, Coping strategies, and spiritual outcomes. *Journal of Religion and Health, 48*(1), 46–57.

National Child Traumatic Stress Network and National Center for PTSD (2005). *Psychological first aid: Field operations guide.* Retrieved 20 Aug 2014 from http://www.vdh.state.va.us/EPR/pdf/PFA9-6-05Final.pdf

Neria, Y., Galea, S., and Norris, F. (Eds) (2009). *Mental Health and Disasters.* New York: Cambridge University Press.

Norris, F. H., Tracy, M., and Galea, S. (2009). Looking for resilience: Understanding the longitudinal trajectories of responses to stress. *Social Science and Medicine, 68*, 2190–2198.

Park, C. L., and Helgeson, V. S. (2006). Introduction to the special section: Growth following highly stressful life events – Current status and future directions. *Journal of Consulting and Clinical Psychology, 74*(5), 791–796.

Paton, D., Smith, L., and Violanti, J. (2000). Disaster response: Risk, vulnerability and resilience. *Disaster Prevention and Management, 9*(3), 173–179. Retrieved 20 Aug 2014 from http://search.proquest.com/docview/214376726?accountid=10382

Phillips, S. B. (2009). The synergy of group and individual treatment modalities in the aftermath of disaster and unfolding trauma. *International Journal of Group Psychotherapy, 59*(1), 85–107.

Pooley, J. A., Cohen, L., O'Connor, M., and Taylor, M. (2012). Posttraumatic stress and posttraumatic growth and their relationship to coping and self-efficacy in Northwest Australian cyclone communities. *Psychological Trauma: Theory Research Practice and Policy, 5*(4), 392–399. doi:10.1037/a0028046

Psychosocial Working Group (PWG) (2003). *Psychosocial intervention in complex emergencies: A framework for practice.* Working Paper, Centre for International Health Studies, Queen Margaret University, Edinburgh.

Rajkumar, A. P., Premkumar, T. S., and Tharyan, P. (2008). Coping with the Asian tsunami: Perspectives from Tamil Nadu, India on the determinants of resilience in the face of adversity. *Social Science and Medicine, 67*(5), 844–853.

Rao, K. (2006). Psychosocial support in disaster-affected communities. *International Review of Psychiatry, 18*(6), 501–505. doi:1237467351.

Romero, P. (2011). *Cultural differences in resilience and coping in ethnic minority populations.* (ProQuest Dissertations and Theses, 197). (Order No. 3478674, Azusa Pacific University). Retrieved 20 Aug 2014 from http://search.proquest.com/docview/903975279?accountid=10382. (903975279).

Rutter, M. (2007). Resilience, competence, and coping. *Child Abuse and Neglect, 31*(3), 205–209.

Saul, J., and Bava, S. (2008). *Implementing collective approaches to massive trauma/loss in western contexts: Implications for recovery, peace building and development.* Paper presented at the Trauma Development and Peace Building Conference, Delhi, India. Retrieved 20 Aug 2014 from http://www.incore.ulst.ac.uk/pdfs/IDRCsaul.pdf

Stellman, J. M., Smith, R. P., Katz, C. L., Sharma, V., Charney, D. S., and Herbert, R. (2008). Enduring mental health morbidity and social function impairment in World Trade Center rescue, recovery, and cleanup workers: The psychological dimension of an environmental health disaster. *Environmental Health Perspectives, 116*(9), 1248–1253.

Strang, A. B., and Ager, A. (2001). *Building a conceptual framework for psychosocial intervention in complex emergencies: Reporting on the work of the Psychosocial Working Group,* 1–6. Centre for International Health Studies, Queen Margaret University, Edinburgh.

Sumathipala, A., and Siribaddana, S. (2005). Research and clinical ethics after the tsunami: Sri Lanka. *The Lancet, 366*(9495), 1418–1420.

Tedeschi, R. G., and Calhoun, L. G. (2004). *Posttraumatic growth: Conceptual foundation and empirical evidence.* Philadelphia, PA: Lawrence Erlbaum Associates.

Vernberg, E. M., Steinberg, A., Jacobs, A., Brymer, M., Watson, P., Osofsky, J., Layne, C. M., Pynoos, R. S., and Ruzek, J. (2008). Innovations in disaster mental health: Psychological first aid. *Professional Psychology – Research and Practice, 39*(4), 381–388.

Vijaykumar, L., Thara, R., John, S., and Chellappa, S. (2006). Psychosocial intervention after tsunami in Tamil Nadu, India. *International Review of Psychiatry, 18*(3), 225–231.

Walsh, F. (2007). Traumatic loss and major disasters: Strengthening family and community resilience. *Family Process, 46*(2), 207–227.

Weingarten, K. (2006). *Compassionate witnessing and the transformation of societal violence: How individuals can make a difference,* 1–21. Retrieved 20 Aug 2014 from http://www.witnessingproject.org/articles/CompassionateWitnessing.pdf

Weinrib, A. Z., Rothrock, N. E., Johnsen, E. L., and Lutgendorf, S. K. (2006). The assessment and validity of stress related growth in a community-based sample. *Journal of Consulting and Clinical Psychology, 74*(5), 851–858.

Winkworth, G. (2007). *Disaster recovery: A review of the literature.* Institute of Child Protection Studies, ACU National, Dixon, ACT. Retrieved 20 Aug 2014 from www.icps@signadou.acu.edu.au

World Health Organization (2005). *WHO framework for mental health and psychosocial support after the tsunami.* Retrieved 20 Aug 2014 from http://www.searo.who.int/LinkFiles/SEA_Earthquake_and_Tsunami_Tsunami_Framework.pdf

World Health Organization, War Trauma Foundation and World Vision International (2011). *Psychological first aid: Guide for field workers.* Retrieved 20 Aug 2014 from http://www.who.int/mental_health/publications/guide_field_workers/en/

Yamazaki, M., Minami, Y., Sasaki, H., and Sumi, M. (2011). The psychosocial response to the 2011 Tohoku earthquake. *Bulletin of the World Health Organization, 89*(9), 623. Retrieved 20 Aug 2014 from http://www.ncbi.nlm.nih.gov/pmc/articles/PMC3165986/

Zoellner, T., Rabe, S., Karl, A., and Maercker, A. (2008). Posttraumatic growth in accident survivors: Openness and optimism as predictors of its constructive or illusory sides. *Journal of Clinical Psychology, 64*(3), 247–261.

Chapter 7

Terrorist attacks, community-level effects, the media and how governments respond

Introduction

Terrorist acts kill and injure many people. There is a ripple of effects that permeate from directly affected victims, to their family members, to their friends and to the wider community. In addition, the rise of the 'citizen journalist' allows the media unprecedented access to such events. As a result there are multiple layers of effects and multiple layers of victims. This chapter discusses the community-level effects of terrorist attacks on different groups in the community, the roles played by the media and, finally, how governments respond.

Background

The 9/11 attacks (2001), the Bali bombings (2002), the Madrid train bombings (2004), the Mumbai attack (2008) and the Israeli–Palestinian experiences (1948 onwards) are all examples of attacks in which terrorism has been used to inflict fear and terror at the individual and community levels. The United States Department of State collates national and international statistics on terrorism (Johnston, 2008): in 2006, at the most recent collation of figures for national and international terrorism, there were 4,981 incidents, 9,175 fatalities and 16,006 injuries. Domestic terrorism contributed significantly to those figures. In Israel alone between September 2000 and January 2006, 7,633 victims were injured in terrorist-related attacks (Tuchner *et al*, 2010).

Part one: community-level effects

The word 'trauma' is used extensively to portray the experience individuals describe when involved in any type of disaster. As discussed previously, research has often concentrated on the effects of a disaster at the individual level, and trauma has often been seen as an unavoidable psychological problem experienced by most victims. Researchers such as Saul and Bava (2008) have moved away from this medical model of trauma at the individual level and have recommended it be viewed as a wider concept which affects not only individuals but families, communities and larger populations, termed 'mass trauma'. Wieling and Mittal (2008) support this notion and suggest there is a gap in the literature regarding the effects of mass trauma at the family and community levels, and that there is even less data on evidence-based interventions to support such victims.

From a trauma perspective, wars such as those experienced in regions such as Syria, Afghanistan, Sri Lanka and the former Yugoslavia produce mass trauma situations where effects are not only experienced at the individual level, but a degree of collective mass trauma is also experienced by the families and people who live in the communities and surrounding districts. A study by Catani, Schauer, and Neuner (2008) examined the consequences of mass trauma in Afghanistan and Sri Lanka, both countries which have endured the consequences of mass trauma and war for long periods of time. The study highlights that many children exposed to prolonged war in countries such as these not only had to endure the effects of mass trauma, but were also exposed to high levels of family violence. These findings have implications for interventions in resource-poor countries in which the population is exposed to war or natural disasters over a long period of time. The suggestion is that interventions need to be tailored to the needs of the wider community and children in a family-centred and culturally appropriate way.

In addition to the study discussed above, a review by Gewirtz, Forgatch, and Wieling (2008) into the mediating effects of parental influences on the effects of trauma in children has been undertaken. This review cites studies undertaken in war zones around the world, such as Cambodia and Israel, where a positive correlation has been found between the mother's level of psychological distress and the extent of the children's PTSD symptoms, recovery and adjustment. It is suggested that interventions which help parents provide a stable. structured environment for their children and which encourage 'security and emotional warmth' will help promote resilience in children exposed to traumatic events (Gewirtz *et al*, 2008, p. 186). In other words, parents' behaviours and reactions will be mirrored and transferred to the children either positively or negatively, depending on the parents' own reactions.

However, the authors consider that the research on this topic has 'languished', with few studies conducted on the correlation between parenting practices and children's adjustment to a major traumatic event. To ameliorate this situation they suggest there is a need for further research which investigates the efficacy of preventative interventions with parents in the aftermath of a mass trauma situation. A psychosocial approach to interventions that considers families, households and communities is likely to fulfil these criteria. The following section examines disaster interventions based on a psychosocial approach to assisting victims.

Impacts on vulnerable groups

Marginalised groups of people are found within most communities and often endure difficulties such as social isolation and economic hardship. Terrorist attacks, as previously discussed, are designed to induce fear in and cause death or injury to as many people as possible. Apart from the difficulties they already experience in the community, the disaster burden following such an attack falls disproportionally on marginalised groups (Eisenman *et al*, 2009). Old age, having a disability, being a teenager, being female, having a mental health problem, being an immigrant or residing in a developing country are all recognised risk factors for being disproportionally affected by disasters (Fjord and Manderson, 2009). The effects on women, older adults and victims with mental health difficulties are discussed in the following sections.

Women and older adults

Ginige, Amaratunga, and Haigh (2009) argue that women are disproportionately affected by disasters, in that they are 'more vulnerable and the most affected by disasters' (p. 23). It is thought this occurs as a direct result of women having less access to resources, and because of their role in fulfilling household duties and providing care for children and elderly relatives (Ginige *et al*, 2009). These direct care roles increase as women have to respond to the situational crises within their households. This in turn leads to more economic hardship within the household, particularly in developing countries, as opportunities for formal and informal employment are often lost (World Bank, n.d.). Women are also disproportionately affected as they experience more mental health problems and mental health conditions (Women's Health Issues, 2009, p. 7), which in many instances will be exacerbated by the disaster.

Older adults are disproportionally affected by disasters of any type. For example, in relation to Hurricane Katrina, a recent study outlined that older adults constituted less than 15 per cent of the population and yet made up 75 per cent of the deceased (Dyer *et al*, 2008). Older adults were disproportionally affected by the 9/11 attacks – there were a large number of older adults living close to the World Trade Center who were traumatised by the events (Jellinek and Willig, 2007). Practical and emotional support of older adults was relatively easy only if they were residents of an aged care facility. If they resided in the community in their own homes there were deficits in the distribution of care in the form of basic necessities for survival. Some older adults were without food, water and essentials for days as care aides were unable to reach them due to damaged infrastructure and security clampdowns. Additionally, deficits in care were seen in those older adults who were unknown to agencies (Jellinek and Willig, 2007).

Wisner comments that marginalisation of vulnerable groups is not just confined to a disaster situation: they experience high levels of harm every day, which disasters then exacerbate (Wisner, cited in Fjord and Manderson, 2009, p. 65). Several studies highlight not only the vulnerability of older adults in human-made and natural disasters, but also the significant deficits in disaster response.

Victims with mental health problems

Most people with a mental health problem can 'benefit from an environment which supports routine, structure, availability of up to date medications and ready access to their mental health professionals' (Milligan and McGuinness, 2009, p. 23). It is likely that, given the effects of terrorist attacks and natural disasters, there will be disruption to most, if not all, of the above stabilising factors. Consequently there is considerable likelihood that victims with previously diagnosed mental health problems will experience an exacerbation of their pre-existing symptoms and illness (Milligan and McGuinness, 2009). Most victims will experience some form of distress even if they have no previous history of mental health problems, so it follows that those with a pre-existing diagnosed mental health problem are more vulnerable in any disaster situation.

Following the Indian Ocean tsunami (2004), the most vulnerable groups were widows, orphans, the aged, disabled and those subjected to discrimination as a result of caste (Sekar *et al*, 2005, p.14). It is likely that in resource-poor countries, individuals with a diagnosed mental health problem would be particularly vulnerable post-attack due to their poor socio-economic circumstances and their minority group status. As well as being particularly vulnerable to exacerbation of their existing mental health difficulties, people with chronic and severe mental illness (SMI) have been shown to have an increased risk of developing PTSD – some 20 to 30 times higher than in the population not experiencing SMI.

Natural or human-made disasters have been positively correlated with the development of PTSD in victims with pre-existing SMI and exacerbating the symptoms of SMI or pre-existing PTSD symptoms (Milligan and McGuinness, 2009). Given these facts, and the distress which victims experience post-attack, it follows that in a post-disaster situation there will be an increase in the uptake and need for psychological services. For example, in the case of Hurricane Katrina, the number of people who presented with a SMI doubled from 6.15 per cent pre-Katrina to 11.3 per cent following the disaster (Calderon-Abbo, 2008). This one disaster particularly highlighted the lack of mental health professionals available to meet the needs of a large group of victims, and informed the basis of a recommendation in chapter 8.

Surprisingly, wars, natural disasters and terrorist attacks have also been shown to be a catalyst for change in mental health services for people with SMI access. As discussed, people with mental health problems are a marginalised and vulnerable group in most societies, and they are likely to experience an exacerbation of symptoms in complex emergencies. In Aceh, Pakistan and Ethiopia, patients presenting with severe mental health disorders outnumbered those with stress-related symptoms (Jones *et al*, 2009). Prior to the disaster, access to mental health services in all these regions was limited. However, in response to the disaster, agencies such as International Medical Corp and the Red Cross entered the area, and as a result there was a corresponding increase in access to services.

An example given by these authors is of a young man in a refugee camp in Darfur who had severe mental health issues and whose family chained him to a tree in the belief it would protect him and those around him from his aggressive psychotic outbursts. The family had fled the conflict zone and brought the young man with them to the camp to seek refuge from the conflict. With appropriate assessment, medication and support from the agencies and his family, the young man's condition improved significantly. This supports the hypothesis that if interventions are readily available and are geared to meet the needs of vulnerable groups, such as those who are separated from their families or children who have lost their parents, progress from the extreme reactions of trauma can be achieved.

Being an older citizen (Eisenman *et al*, 2009), having mental health problems (Milligan and McGuinness, 2009) and living in a resource-poor country (Catani *et al*, 2008) are all factors that predispose these marginalised groups of people to shouldering a disproportionate level of the disaster burden (Eisenman *et al*, 2009). It is therefore clear that in any type of disaster, older adults and other marginalised groups need to be given priority in the various stages of response and should be listed as a priority in strategic disaster plans. Due to the paucity of studies which examine the effects of disaster on vulnerable groups, there is a need for further research in this area.

The community support approach

As indicated, communities and their residents play an important part in post-disaster recovery, as that is where individuals and groups return in the post-disaster recovery phase. Governments and funding bodies are now recognising the importance of communities in post-disaster mitigation. India is particularly vulnerable to natural disasters, with millions of people affected on an annual basis by cyclones, floods, droughts and landslides (Indian Red Cross Society, n.d). This results in high numbers of fatalities and injured, with many left homeless as their homes are destroyed, swept away or damaged beyond repair.

Recognising the importance of communities, a global initiative – the Community Disaster Resilience Fund (CDRF) – uses schemes to direct funds to vulnerable communities to enhance their disaster-preparedness. It is vital that communities and agencies are ready and prepared to respond in a complex emergency, as it is posited that the responses and decisions made in the first 72 hours of an emergency will 'lay the foundation for an effective emergency response in the following six to eight weeks' (UNICEF, p. 4, n.d.).

Such schemes operate in India, where funds are given to eight organisations operating in 88 villages in seven states prone to natural disasters (Gopalan, n.d.). The schemes are designed to enhance preparedness for disasters and build community resilience. Each community is required to collaborate and produce an action plan to identify needs in the case of a disaster such as a flood or cyclone. Vulnerable and disaster-prone areas are identified, as well as safe areas to which people can quickly move. Additionally, villagers most at risk, such as the sick, women and children, are acknowledged. Villagers can move to a safe area as soon as a cyclone is forecast, and the vulnerable are supported to do the same. Four similar grassroots women-led Community Disaster Resilience pilots are also underway in Latin America (Gopalan, n.d.).

This community support approach was also put to good use post-disaster in India following the 2004 tsunami and included community self-help groups, relaxation exercises and the use of cultural metaphors to help the victims come to terms with their experience (Becker, 2009, Bonanno *et al*, 2007). Some problems were experienced in the rebuilding phases of the response, however, given the need to rehouse the many thousands left homeless by the disaster. In Tamil Nadu a few of the communities banded together to garner the support they required. They were communities who had pre-existing strong social bonds and social capital and appeared to receive aid and support from external agencies quite quickly; this was because they were able to prepare beforehand and voice what was needed for recovery very well. They did this using pre-existing organised community elders and representatives, who produced a clear written list of needs soon after the tsunami hit. This was a case of a community being well informed and well prepared prior to a disaster.

Disquiet arose elsewhere when villagers who had lost their homes and who had lived and fished by the ocean all their lives, and made their livelihood from it, were relocated away from the ocean – they objected to this, and it resulted in them feeling they had been overlooked in the recovery and decision-making process (Raju, 2013).

In Australia, jointly funded state and Commonwealth projects such as the Natural Disaster Resilience Program (NDRP) have been initiated to promote community preparedness and resilience through funding of particular programmes such as the Emergency Volunteer Support Scheme, State Emergency Management Projects, the Auxiliary Disaster Resilience Grants Scheme, the Bush Fire Risk Management Grants Scheme and the Floodplain Risk Management Grants Scheme (New South Wales Government State Emergency Plan, 2012).

Summary

Disaster does not discriminate, and those who are vulnerable are at most risk. Older members of society, the disabled, those with a mental health problem and those who are socially disadvantaged are at the greatest risk of death or injury. Current research suggests that if interventions are readily available and are geared to meet the needs of vulnerable and marginalised groups, their propensity to carry a disproportionate weight of the disaster burden can be greatly reduced. Ultimately the risk for all communities can be reduced if funding is aimed at preparing communities for disasters, with targeted programmes in disaster-prone areas which aim to enhance the community's readiness and resilience pre and post-disaster.

Part two: television and social media

The media are an important medium for bringing news of all types to the public. Few can forget the graphic images of the 9/11 attacks as the aeroplanes were deliberately flown into the Twin Towers in New York. In Bali a number of victims reported that the television and newspaper coverage of the attack was extremely graphic (personal communication, February 2008). A new television station had just commenced broadcasting when the attack occurred, and was on the scene and at the main hospital very soon after the attack. It was reported that very graphic and bloody scenes were filmed at the bombing site and the hospital without any noticeable degree of censorship. Normal coverage was interrupted to show live coverage from the hospital and bombing site, which was reportedly seen by many children.

These graphic scenes would have added to the children's considerable distress; it is also now recognised that victims who were not directly exposed to critical incidents but who have viewed them on television or in print may also present with longer lasting distress symptoms, such as depression, nightmares and anxiety (Dougall *et al*, 2005; Park *et al*, 2008; Propper *et al*, 2007).

As previously noted, children's distress and fear as a result of these factors is evident from their parents' descriptions. In one instance described by an interviewee the child was still afraid in 2008, some six years after the bombing; another's distress continued for three years.

> My daughter [7 in 2002] [was] afraid every time she watch[ed] TV and saw a show about criminal[s] and dead people. [After] the bomb blast [was] she quiet for a month; didn't want to play or eat; she was really trauma[tised].
> (Wife of injured male)

> His mental state became really down. He didn't want to go out; he was afraid with people and afraid when the lights went out [this continued for three years].
> (Injured female victim, commenting on the effects on her son, aged six)

In contemporary society, Facebook, Twitter, personal blogs, Skype, Flickr, digital photographs and uploaded video images are all methods most of us use to communicate with and share information with our peers online on a daily basis. The use of social media in most countries is high and in the United States 65 per cent of adult internet users are said to use such sites as a form of social interaction (Thackeray *et al*, 2012). This rise of social media is changing the ways in which news is disseminated and read. Since the 9/11 attacks and the Bali bombings, forms of reporting everyday general news and terrorist attacks have changed.

Citizen journalists abound, especially during disasters, as people turn to their phones and computers to record the events. During the London bombings the events as they unfolded were recorded and disseminated by men and women who were caught up in the events. The role of citizen journalist was described by Allan (cited in Downman, 2013, p.154) as involving 'spontaneous actions of ordinary people compelled to adopt the role of a journalist in order to bear witness to what is happening'.

One of the most prolific examples of citizen journalists' reporting of terrorist activities was seen during the Mumbai attacks of November 2008, in which a group of men attacked eight sites around Mumbai with handheld weapons and bombs. The attacks killed 173 people and left 293 injured (Javaid and Kamal, 2013). The attacks were unique as they took place over a three-day period and were reported almost minute-by-minute through accounts relayed on television news, Facebook, Twitter, personal blogs, Skype, Flickr and uploaded digital photographs, video images and newspapers. News and images were delivered instantly to the internet for local and international viewing (Bianco, 2009).

As print media readership declines, social media appears to be replacing it. This form of almost instant communication brings the news as it happens, with even news organisations constantly tweeting their headlines (Zeichek, cited in Murthy, 2009). However, little editing appears to be carried out by citizen journalists and this can result in graphic images being relayed into global audiences' living rooms, with the same potential for vicarious trauma previously discussed. It also gives the terrorists the attention and publicity they desire, enabling them to bring fear to the people and communities they attack but also to the many others who are watching the events unfold across the world. In Mumbai it was also determined that the terrorists monitored the same forms of professional and social media to manipulate the news, plan their attacks and communicate with their handlers back in Pakistan (Desai and Dharurkar, 2012).

Summary

As a result of the issues discussed above, there is debate as to the role played by the media in terms of reconfiguring disasters, shaping how the world sees them and establishing and re-establishing the forces that gave birth to disasters in the first place (Cottle, 2014). Desai and Dharurkar (2012) strongly make the case for responsible and ethical media reporting and for journalists to set out a clear demarcation between ethical and unethical journalism. While it is argued that news media self-regulation is working in some countries, it may be time to look at developing the research in this fast-changing area.

Part three: how do governments respond?

Terrorism is designed to instil fear and panic in the communities attacked, and governments will often respond to allay the fears of the general public at the earliest time possible. Due to the complexities of government policies, public opinions and legislative powers, there is no 'one size fits all' response that governments will use. While the Australian and Indonesian responses to the 2002 bombings in Bali are the main focus of this section, the British and American responses to terrorist attacks are also outlined.

Response to the Bali bombing

Three years prior to the bombings, the number of Australians taking their holidays overseas had been predicted to continue to increase annually (Robins *et al*, 1999). In the aftermath of the bombing the Australian government immediately responded with a travel advisory issued through the media and the official Department of Foreign Affairs and Trade (DFAT) web site (DFAT, 2002). The advisory strongly discouraged Australians from travelling to all areas of Indonesia due to the high risk of future terrorist activity (Hill, 2002). Interestingly, a visit to the travel advisory website in December 2013 saw a similar advisory listed (DFAT, 2013), and in January 2014 it was recommended that the traveller exercise a high degree of caution (DFAT, 2014).

The bombings and government warnings post-attack had a detrimental effect on tourism to the region, with many Australians cancelling pre-booked holidays to Bali or deciding not to book their traditional annual holiday to the region. Instead, travellers chose other destinations overseas or decided to take their annual holiday in Australia, where they felt safer. These decisions contributed to a stronger domestic travel season, with places like Queensland benefiting from an increased domestic tourist market which saw a return to positive growth in 2002 (Queensland Government, 2002). Other governments, such as those of Canada, the United States and Japan, issued general travel warnings to their nationals regarding travel to Southeast Asia, adding to the large downturn of tourism in the region. Aside from the downturns in international tourism seen in Australia and Indonesia, other countries in the region experienced a similar effect, reportedly as a direct result of the travel warnings issued by Australia and other foreign governments.

Co-operation across countries

The 2002 bombings had an immediate effect, with Australia and America among a number of other western countries revisiting previous calls for Indonesia to crack down on militant Islamic groups. In an eight-page document issued on 22 October 2002, 11 days following the bombing, Dr Stephen Sherlock of the Australian Department of Foreign Affairs, Defence and Trade made a statement in which he heavily criticised the Indonesian government's policy on Islamic extremist groups, as well as corruption in the legal system, their policy on official corruption, economic stagnation, separatist conflicts, communal violence and the credibility of the military (Sherlock, 2002). This was potentially quite an inflammatory statement considering that there appeared to be little evidence to support the standpoint, and given that Australia was trying to nourish a good political relationship with Indonesia at the time.

Surprisingly, despite the level of criticism aimed at Indonesia, evidence indicates its authorities worked well with the Australian government, Australian federal police and the Australian Defence Force. Shortly after the bombings, the Australian and Indonesian authorities formed a joint investigative task force formed from senior members of the Australian and Indonesian federal police. This increased co-operation and sharing of knowledge and information led to the 'identification and arrest of most of those who took part in the attack' (DFAT, 2004).

Equally, operation 'Bali Assist' (Hampson *et al*, 2002), which took place in the aftermath of the bombing, required the co-operation of the Indonesian police, medical and airport authorities to help with the logistics of establishing a field hospital in a hangar at Denpasar airport, where Australian evacuees were stabilised prior to their flight back to Australia. The evacuation of injured Australian citizens was quickly facilitated, with Australian Defence Force Hercules transport planes, civilian medical retrieval flights and Qantas planes landing at Denpasar airport to evacuate the injured within 24 hours of the bombing. Three evacuation flights took place over a period of 21 hours (Hampson *et al*, 2002).

Counter-terrorism measures

Partly as a result of the Bali bombing and the events of 9/11, Australia signed a number of counter-terrorism agreements with other countries in the region, including Indonesia and Malaysia. The agreements represented an effort to combat terrorism and terrorism-related activities both inside and outside Australia's borders. The agreements related to joint intelligence and sharing of information, and Michaelsen (2004, p. 322) suggests that they 'strengthened cooperation between law enforcement agencies'. The 9/11 attack in America was the catalyst that spurred the Australian government into action, as it realised that Australia was also vulnerable to future terrorist attacks.

Several bills were introduced into parliament in March 2002 (seven months prior to the Bali bombings) which specifically related to anti-terrorism laws (Williams, 2002). The bills passed the legislative process in July 2002. They included tighter border control laws, financial regulatory procedures (designed to detect illegal monetary transfers), amendments to the telecommunications act (which saw an increased availability of interception warrants) and a strengthening of laws to protect critical infrastructure such as energy, utilities, health and food supplies (Williams, 2002).

Additional laws related to 'tighter aviation and border control measures' were designed to help ensure passenger safety and bolster consumer confidence in travel (Michaelsen, 2004, p. 322). The legislation required all airlines to send passenger details to immigration and customs in advance, to enable checks against alert lists for passengers entering and leaving Australia. Customs now undertakes risk analysis and profiling of passengers entering Australia through airports (Australian Customs and Border Protection Annual Report 2009–10). According to Michaelsen (2004, p. 334), 'never before in history has Australia witnessed a comparable overhaul of laws that significantly curtailed civil liberties and fundamental freedoms'. Michaelsen accuses the Howard government of a 'clear over reaction', presumably because he had previously concluded there was a 'low risk of attack occurring on Australian soil' (Michaelsen, 2004, p. 321). To date this assumption can be considered correct, as there have been no terrorist attacks in Australia.

To support the legislative steps outlined above and other measures, the Commonwealth government significantly increased the security budget. Following September 2001, the budget was increased by A\$2.3 billion (over a five-year period), specifically to fund additional federal and state security measures. This was followed with another A\$754.5 million in the 2004–2005 budget, bringing the total increase in the security budget over an eight-year period to A\$39.7 billion (Australian Government, 2004). Due to this larger than usual allocation of funds, pressure was exerted on other Commonwealth and state budgets and funds were diverted away from other projects (DFAT, 2004).

The government response in England

In England, the Terrorism Act was issued by the then Labour government and was designed to increase police power to stop, arrest and detain suspects. An insight into the extensive power given to the police at that time was demonstrated by the fact that Article 5 of the European Rights Campaign, promoting the rights to liberty of all citizens and the right to a fair trial, was completely removed. This meant that citizens who were suspected of terrorist activities with little evidence or who were suspected of being members of terrorist groups could be lawfully detained without trial for an indefinite period. The legislation bore similarities to that set in America in response to the 9/11 attacks (HMSO, 2001).

The American response

Following the 9/11 attack, the American government led by Republican President Bush declared a 'war on terrorism': an armed response primarily aimed at eliminating militant organisations, particularly Al Qaeda and its leader Osama bin Laden, who were believed to be responsible for 9/11 and other attacks. This was an example of a government taking steps to calm its citizens and to be seen as taking a tough response to the largest terrorist attack and subsequent loss of life experienced on American soil. The United States, the United Kingdom, Pakistan and many other nations took part in the global response in an effort to combat the rise of transnational terrorism. The United States invaded Iraq in 2003 with the avowed intention of assisting Iraq to become a democracy as part of the American-inspired 'Global War on Terrorism' (Heinze, 2011).

Within America, as in England, the police were given wide-reaching powers to monitor citizens' telephone calls and emails, as well as to detain people indefinitely without the usual parameters set within the law. Merely suspecting someone to be a member of a terrorist group was enough to see them detained indefinitely without the usual process of trial by jury and the right to a defence. On 13 November 2001 a unique order was signed by President Bush which meant any non-US citizen merely suspected of being a terrorist, even should there be little or no evidence, could be removed from the usual jurisdiction of the criminal courts and instead tried by specially convened military commissions with their own set of military laws (Patriot Act, 2001).

Hundreds of people who were deemed unlawful 'enemies of the state' were then transferred to Guantanamo Bay, a remote camp in Cuba set up specifically to hold such prisoners. The prisoners in Guantanamo Bay were shackled and often hooded to ensure sensory deprivation and, once arrived, were imprisoned in wire mesh cages (Amnesty International, 2012). President Bush signed an order later in 2001 decreeing that none of the detainees would be classified as prisoners of war or governed by the 1949 Geneva Convention Article 3, which forbids humiliating or degrading treatment. In other words, the law protecting prisoners from inhumane treatment was withdrawn.

It took only two years for the International Human Rights commission to comment on the deteriorating psychological health of a number of the detainees (http://www.amnesty.ca/our-work/issues/security-and-human-rights/ guantanamo-bay). In 2009 President Obama promised to close the facilities, yet in 2012 the president of the International Human Rights Commission, Navi Pilla, criticised the government for not having done so and for passing a new act, the National Defense Authorization Act (NDAA), which allows for the indefinite detention without trial of certain citizens (UN News, 2012), thereby continuing the abuse of human rights. With 150 men still detained at Guatanamo, Amnesty International has recently called for an 'impartial investigation into what it suggests are credible allegations of human rights violations in Guantanamo' (Amnesty International, 2014, p. 1).

Summary

Governments have a right to respond when their citizens are attacked on home or foreign soil. Lessons can and should be learned from the global response to terrorism, and we see a concerted effort to do this post 9/11. These lessons add to the body of literature that maps human and societal responses to what are very complex situations for all.

Terrorist attacks have been part of our global society for thousands of years and impact every level of society. With the development of social media and the ability of individuals to impact the process, outcome and aftermath of complex emergencies, governments charged with the responsibility to deal with these situations are often in a very difficult position. Contemporary responses to terrorists see governments starting to work together internationally, beyond their national policies and strategies, which may ultimately assist in defusing some of the reasons for the attacks in the first place.

References

Amnesty International (2012). *Guantanamo Bay: Get the Facts*. Retrieved 20 Aug 2014 from http://www.amnesty.org.au/hrs/comments

Amnesty International (2014). *Iraq: Security failures raise fears of election violence*. Retrieved 20 Aug 2014 from https://www.amnesty.org/en/news/iraq-security-failures-raise-fears-election-violence-2014-04-29

Her Majesty's Stationery Office (HMSO), The National Archives (2001). Antiterrorism crime and security act. 2001 Chapter 24. Retrieved 20 Aug 2014 from http://www.legislation.gov.uk/ukpga/2001/24/contents

Australian Customs and Border Protection Annual Report (2009–10). *Border Risk 9: Airline Security*. Retrieved 20 Aug 2014 from http://www.customs.gov.au/webdata/minisites/annualreport0809/pages/page115.html

Australian Government (2004). *Budget at a glance (2004–2005)*. Retrieved 20 Aug 2014 from http://www.budget.gov.au/2004-05/at_a_glance/download/budget_at_a_glance.pdf

Becker, S. (2009). Psychosocial care for women survivors of the tsunami disaster in India. *American Journal of Public Health, 99*(4), 654–658. doi:10.2105/AJPH.2008.146571

Bianco, J. S. (2009). Social networking and cloud computing: Precarious affordances for the 'prosumer'. *Women's Studies Quarterly, 37*, 303–312.

Bonanno, G. A., Galea, S., Bucciarelli, A., and Vlahov, D. (2007). What predicts psychological resilience after disaster? The role of demographics, resources, and life stress. *Journal of Consulting and Clinical Psychology, 75*(5), 671–682.

Calderon-Abbo, J. (2008). The long road home: Rebuilding public inpatient psychiatric services in post-Katrina New Orleans. *Psychiatric Services, 59*(3), 304–308.

Catani, C., Schauer, E., and Neuner, F. (2008). Beyond individual war trauma: Domestic violence against children in Afghanistan and Sri Lanka. *Journal of Marital and Family Therapy, 34*(2), 166–173.

Cottle, S. (2014). Rethinking media and disasters in a global age: What's changed and why it matters. *Media, War and Conflict, 7*(1), 3–22.

Department of Foreign Affairs and Trade (DFAT) (2002, 15 October). *Travel advice, Indonesia*. Retrieved 20 Aug 2014 from http://www.smartraveller.gov.au/zw-egi/view/Advice/Indonesia

Department of Foreign Affairs and Trade (DFAT) (2004). *Transnational terrorism: The threat to Australia. Chapter 2: A new kind of foe*. Information sheet 5. Retrieved 20 Aug 2014 from http://www.dfat.gov.au/publications/terrorism/chapter2.html

Department of Foreign Affairs and Trade (DFAT) (2013, 10 January). *Travel advice, Indonesia*. Retrieved 20 Aug 2014 from http://www.smartraveller.gov.au/zw-cgi/view/Advice/Indonesia

Department of Foreign Affairs and Trade (DFAT) (2014, 5 January). *Travel advice, Indonesia*. Retrieved 20 Aug 2014 from http://smartraveller.gov.au/zw-cgi/view/Advice/Indonesia

Desai, G., and Dharurkar, V. L. (2012). Understanding effect of mass media on disaster management: A case study. *International Journal of Research in Social Sciences, 2*(1), 127–132. Retrieved 20 Aug 2014 from http://search.proquest.com/docview/1011564396?accountid=10382

Dougall, A. L., Hayward, M. C., and Baum, A. (2005). Media exposure to bioterrorism: Stress and the anthrax attacks. *Psychiatry: Interpersonal and Biological Processes, 68*(1), 28–42.

Downman, S. (2013). Reporting disasters from inside a repressive regime: A citizen journalism case study of the 2008 Cyclone Nargis disaster. *Australian Journal of Communication, 40*(1), 153–172. Retrieved 20 Aug 2014 from http://search.proquest.com/docview/1450264660?accountid=10382

Dyer, C. B., Regev, M., Burnett, J., Festa, N., and Cloyd, B. (2008). SWiFT: A rapid triage tool for vulnerable older adults in disaster situations. *Disaster Medicine and Public Preparedness, 29*(1), s45–s50.

Eisenman, D. P., Glik, D., Ong, M., Zhou, Q., Tseng, C., Long, A., Fielding, J., and Asch, S. (2009). Terrorism-related fear and avoidance behavior in a multiethnic urban population. *American Journal of Public Health, 99*(1), 168–174.

Fjord, L., and Manderson, L. (2009). Anthropological perspectives on disasters and disability: An introduction. *Human Organization, 68*(1), 64–72. Retrieved 20 Aug 2014 from http://search.proquest.com/docview/201171341?accountid=10382

Gewirtz, A., Forgatch, M., and Wieling, E. (2008). Parenting practices as potential mechanisms for child adjustment following mass trauma. *Journal of Marital and Family Therapy, 34*(2), 177–187.

Ginige, K., Amaratunga, D., and Haigh, R. (2009). Mainstreaming gender in a disaster reduction: why and how. *Disaster Prevention and Management, 18*(1), 23–34.

Gopalan, P. (n.d.). Huairou Commission Delegation Statement. Retrieved 20 Aug 2014 from http://www.google.com.au/url?sa=t&rct=j&q=&esrc=s&source=web&cd=2&ved=0CDAQFjAB&url=http%3A%2F%2Fwww.preventionweb.net%2Ffiles%2Fglobalplatform%2FPlenaryStatementHCPrema.doc&ei=8ihfU__LJIimkwXo2ICACQ&usg=AFQjCNFu6K8sQ9JDLg7y7-YRXVUV0eNy9w

Hampson, G. V., Cook, S. P., and Frederiksen, S. R. (2002). Operation Bali Assist: The Australian defence force response to the Bali bombing. *The Medical Journal of Australia, 177*(11/12), 620–623.

Heinze, E. A. (2011). The evolution of international law in light of the 'global war on terror'. *Review of International Studies, 37*(3), 1069–1094. doi:http://dx.doi.org/10.1017/S0260210510001014

Hill, R. (2002, 14 October). *Senator Hill's speech on the Bali bombings.* Retrieved 20 Aug 2014 from http://australianpolitics.com/news/2002/10/02-10-14b

Indian Red Cross Society (n.d.). *India: Community-based disaster risk reduction programme.* Retrieved 20 Aug 2014 from http://www.indianredcross.org/publications/community-based-disaster-risk-reduction%20Programme-Maharashtra.pdf

Javaid, U., and Kamal, M. (2013). The Mumbai terror 2008 and its impact on the Indo-Pak relations. *South Asian Studies, 28*(1), 25–37. Retrieved 20 Aug 2014 from http://search.proquest.com/docview/1369670732?accountid=10382

Jellinek, I., and Willig, J. (2007). When a terrorist attacks: September 11 and the impact on older adults in New York City. *Generations, 31*(4), 42–46.

Johnston, W. R. (2008). *Statistics on international terrorism.* Retrieved 20 Aug 2014 from http://www.johnstonsarchive.net/terrorism/intlterror.html

Jones, L., Asare, J. B., El Masri, M., Mohanraj, A., Sherief, H., and Van Ommeren, M. (2009). Severe mental disorders in complex emergencies. *The Lancet, 374*, 654–661.

Michaelsen, C. (2004). Antiterrorism legislation in Australia: A proportionate response to the terrorist threat. *Studies in Conflict and Terrorism, 28*, 321–339.

Milligan, G., and McGuinness, T. M. (2009). Mental health needs in a post-disaster environment. *Journal of Psychosocial Nursing and Mental Health Services, 47*(9), 23–30.

Murthy, D. (2009). *Understanding some policy implications of Twitter*. Department of Sociology, Bowdoin College. Retrieved 20 Aug 2014 from http://www.lse.ac.uk/media@lse/events/MeCCSA/pdf/papers/MURTHY_LSE%20media%20and%20communication%20policy%20paper.pdf

NSW State Emergency Management Plan (2012) Retrieved 20 Aug 2014 from http://www.emergency.nsw.gov.au/media/1621.pdf

Park, C. L., Aldwin, C. M., Fenster, J. R., and Snyder, L. B. (2008). Pathways to posttraumatic growth versus posttraumatic stress: Coping and emotional reactions following the September 11, 2001 terrorist attacks. *American Journal of Orthopsychiatry, 78*(3), 300–312.

The Patriot Act (2001). Retrieved 20 Aug 2014 from http://www.gpo.gov/fdsys/pkg/BILLS-107hr3162enr/pdf/BILLS-107hr3162enr.g

Propper, R. E., Stickgold, R., Keeley, R., and Christman, S. D. (2007). Is television traumatic? Dreams, stress, and media exposure in the aftermath of September 11, 2001. *Psychological Science, 18*(4), 334–340.

Queensland Government (2002). *Proposed regulation of tourism services in Queensland. Public Benefit Test report.* Retrieved 20 Aug 2014 from http://ncp.ncc.gov.au/docs/Qld%20proposed%20regulation%20of%20tourism%20services%20-%20PBT.pdf

Raju, E. (2013). Housing reconstruction in disaster recovery: A study of fishing communities post-tsunami in Chennai, India. *PLoS Current Disasters*, Apr 3. Edition 1. doi:10.1371/currents.dis.a4f34a96cb91aaffacd36f5ce7476a36

Robins, P., Hamal, K., and Rosetto, A. (1999). Australian tourism outlook. *Proceedings of the Australian Tourism Outlook Conference*, 1–22. Retrieved 20 Aug 2014 from http://www.ret.gov.au/tourism/Documents/tra/Snapshots%20and%20Factsheets/99.5%20Australian%20Tourism%20Outlook.pdf

Saul, J., and Bava, S. (2008). Implementing collective approaches to massive trauma/loss in western contexts: Implications for recovery, peace building and development. Paper presented at the Trauma Development and Peace Building Conference, Delhi, India. Retrieved 20 Aug 2014 from http://www.incore.ulst.ac.uk/pdfs/IDRCsaul.pdf

Sekar, K., Biswas, G., Bhadra, S., Jayakumar, C., and Kumar, K. (2005). *Tsunami – Psychosocial care for children*. Bangalore, New Delhi: National Institute of Mental Health and Neuroscience, Care India.

Sherlock, S. (2002, 22 October). The Bali bombing: What it means for Indonesia. Parliament of Australia, Parliamentary Library. *Current Issues Brief 2002–2003(4)*. Retrieved 20 Aug 2014 from http://www.aph.gov.au/library/pubs/cib/2002–03/03cib04.pdf

Thackeray, R., Neiger, B. L., Smith, A. K., and Van Wagenen, S. B. (2012). Adoption and use of social media among public health departments. *BMC Public Health, 12*, 242. doi:http://dx.doi.org/10.1186/1471-2458-12-242

Tuchner, M., Meiner, Z., Parush, S., and Hartman-Maeir, A. (2010). Relationships between sequelae of injury, participation, and quality of life in survivors of terrorist attacks. *OTJR: Occupation, Participation and Health, 30*(1), 29–36.

UN News Centre (2012). *UN Rights chief speaks out against US failure to close Guantanamo detention facility.* Retrieved 20 Aug 2014 from http://www.un.org/apps/news/story. asp?NewsID=41001&Cr=prison&Cr1=rights#.U1_GYYXyWrw

UNICEF (n.d.). *UNICEF emergency field handbook. A guide for UNICEF staff.* http:// www.unicef.org/lac/emergency_handbook.pdf

Wieling, E., and Mittal, M. (2008). JMFT special section on mass trauma. *Journal of Marital and Family Therapy, 34*(2), 127–131.

Williams, D. Hon. (2002, 4 June). *Counter terrorism package.* Retrieved 20 Aug 2014 from http://parlinfo.aph.gov.au/parlInfo/search/display/display.w3p;query=%28Id: media/pressrel/6gp66%29;rec=0

Women's Health Issues (2009). *Women and violence.* Women's Health Victoria. Retrieved 20 Aug 2014 from http://www.whv.org.au/publications-resources/issues-papers

World Bank (n.d.). *The handbook for estimating the socio-economic and environmental effects of disasters,* 1–11. Retrieved 20 Aug 2014 from http://siteresources.worldbank.org/ INTDISMGMT/Resources/10women.pdf

A post-disaster planning framework – opportunities for multidisciplinary application

Introduction

Terrorist attacks frighten, intimidate and cause large-scale injury to civilians. During the response to any type of disaster, governments will turn to professionals who they assume will have the expertise to help in the immediate aftermath of a crisis. In most countries this will include health practitioners, government and non-government agencies. It is likely that many individuals, professionals and organisations will have a viewpoint as to what type of support is required following attacks and natural disasters. This study focused on the experiences reported by primary-level victims, their family members and first responders in the immediate aftermath of the attack and up to six years later.

Although this book focuses on the 2002 Bali terrorist attack, the recommendations are primarily aimed at agencies that plan for the aftermath of such an attack; however, they can be generalised and used by agencies involved in planning for any type of complex emergency. The recommendations are derived from in-depth analysis of the participant interviews, researchers' observations, an in-depth review of the literature and grey data, and draw on the findings of the study.

The Bali disaster revealed the strength of human spirit and resilience and the willingness of people and countries to help each other in times of extreme distress. It also highlighted aspects of the response which could be improved. It is recognised that each disaster is unique, with different effects and requirements for support (Larson *et al*, 2006), and therefore a single response framework may not fit all response requirements; there is thus a need to contextualise according to the needs of each complex emergency. It is also imperative in any complex crisis that rescue and support interventions must take into account the setting, culture and context of the event.

For many people in the immediate vicinity of a disaster, the first response is a desire to help. There will be a structured official response from professional organisations such as the police, fire brigade and ambulance service, as well as an informal unofficial response by way of volunteers. There has to be some means by which professional organisations can work together in an ordered and, where possible, planned manner. The findings of this study revealed multiple layers of effects.

Depleted resources, including sleeplessness, confusion, nightmares and anger, are experienced by up to 90 per cent of terrorist attack survivors (Trappler, 2010). Most of these distressful effects can be termed normal distress reactions to a very abnormal event and, unless these symptoms last longer than a month (Vijaykumar *et al*, 2006), they would be viewed by most mental health practitioners as normal.

It is recognised that there are groups who endure a disproportionate share of a disaster burden (Fjord and Manderson, 2009): these include women, children, the elderly and people with disabilities. Addressing this inequality has to be a priority in responses to any disaster situation. Children were particularly affected by the events in Bali as, apart from potentially hearing the explosions and witnessing the devastation and injuries to family members, they were also exposed to graphic images of the aftermath of the bombing relayed on the television and directly into their homes without any noticeable degree of censorship (personal communication, 2008).

In terms of support or reinforced resources, a large proportion of support comes from immediate family members and friends. Overall, the importance of practical, economic and spiritual support cannot be overlooked. Positive social support in the form of empathetic discussions, basic food supplies, money, childcare and help during elaborate burial ceremonies was an important part of the support in Bali. Given findings of a pre-existing 'pool of resources' (PWG, 2003, p. 2) in most communities, victims must be given help and encouragement to enable them to tap into local support as soon as possible after any major catastrophic event. This type of support is seen as crucial to an individual's recovery, as a sense of 'communal openness' evolves which can help mediate the effects of a disaster (Steury *et al*, 2004), decrease the individual's depression levels, and has been correlated with an increase in levels of resilience (Moscardino *et al*, 2010). The PWG suggests any external agencies that respond to help in an emergency situation should take into account the pre-existing resources within a community. It also suggests that the external support community 'collaborates and negotiates' with the affected community, particularly in developing countries (PWG, p. 2), so that culturally relevant and efficient interventions can occur.

In our everyday interactions we try to achieve a state of emotional, physical and social stability. Terrorist attacks challenge and disrupt this state of stability. As a result, in emergencies there is a 'complex interplay between protection threats and issues of mental health and psychosocial wellbeing' (Inter-Agency Standing Committee, 2006, p. 32). The term 'psychosocial well-being' has been explained as involving 'social, cultural and psychological influences on wellbeing' (PWG, p. 1). The multilayered effects of terrorist attacks and the post-attack support in the Bali situation were examined within a psychosocial framework which encompassed the following domains:

- human capacity, namely the skills and knowledge of people;
- social capacity, namely familial, religious and cultural resources;
- culture and values, namely cultural values, beliefs and practices.

In this book, the physical and psychological effects on victims have been well documented. However, external factors, such as the loss of a job or being unable to work, can cause victims additional socio-economic hardship. There may also be widespread external disruption to the victims' communities with roads, electricity and water supplies disrupted for many days, as occurred following the Asian tsunami and the Fukushima nuclear disaster in Japan.

As resources within domains are disrupted, the PWG (2003, p. 2) suggest there is a 'pool of resources' within the same domains which can be utilised by communities and individuals in response to such emergencies. For example, human capacity may be engaged to promote social linkage, culture and values (PWG, 2003). The effectiveness with which the individual and community utilise these resources may indicate the extent of their adjustment and resilience to the situation.

The aim of using this framework to study the Bali bombings was to detail the 'nature and impact of the event and circumstances' (Strang and Ager, 2001, p. 4) in Bali and Perth. The questions within the in-depth interviews were based around this framework and helped gain valuable knowledge and insight into the multilayered effects of the bombing, the multi-layered support the victims received and the pool of resources utilised by victims and their communities in the aftermath of the bombings. The modified PWG framework developed in this study and the recommendations that emerged from the findings are presented in the next sections of this chapter.

The modified framework

A modified framework based on the 'Framework for Practice' working paper produced by Strang and Ager (2001) will be outlined. The modified framework generated by the findings in this study has been produced for agencies who may wish to develop a strategic and psychosocial approach to disaster planning. It is also intended for use when there is a need to choose appropriate and culturally relevant post-disaster interventions. It is based on the premise, as demonstrated in the experiences documented in this study, that the unexpected can, and does, happen; when it does, it is important for organisations to be prepared and ready to respond and manage the hazards to prevent unnecessary loss of life, injury or distress and reduce the time it takes for the community to recover and improve post-event decision-making (Hollis, 2007).

This framework is not intended to replace a needs analysis or a comprehensive plan for a disaster response. It is purely a framework and starting point upon which organisations may wish to base their strategic plans and initial response strategies. Use of this framework will inform planners and allow them to forecast the possible impact of a disaster through the lenses of human capacity, social ecology and culture and values. Through the same domains lies a framework for disaster response which will accommodate needs which vary in accordance with organisational, geographic and cultural areas.

Broad outlines are given with reference to the domains listed purely to illustrate how the framework can be utilised pre- and post-disaster. As discussed previously, when a disaster such as a terrorist attack occurs, the stock of pre-existing resources at the individual and community levels are depleted. When formulating a response plan it is important for the relevant agencies to assess what resources pre-exist in the local community, what may be utilised by the community in response and where there may be shortfalls. Any psychosocial response to a disaster must consider collaboration and inclusion of the local community within its disaster plan and intervention approaches. This is because communities form an essential part of a contemporary approach to preparedness in a disaster and become part of a process in which regional knowledge can be utilised and nuances can be addressed (El Haq, 2007).

It is posited within this study and framework that the immediate needs of disaster victims are best assessed and planned for initially under the domain of human capacity, as there is a rich and reinforcing set of resources available within the community for support in the aftermath of a disaster. Human capacity is described by the PWG (2003, p. 2) as 'the physical and mental needs of the community members, their existing skills and knowledge and their household livelihoods'. The remaining domains of social ecology and culture and values are also important factors to be considered in assessing the possible impacts of a disaster. Social ecology refers to the social capital of a community, such as families, peer groups, religious groups and civil and political authorities, while culture and values refers to the cultural capital of a community, such as its cultural beliefs and practices (Strang and Ager, 2001, p. 3). Within this framework the domains are interrelated and are discussed in terms of disrupted and reinforced resources. When utilised and where appropriate they are highlighted in brackets.

The framework is illustrated in Figure 8.1, which is followed by a discussion illustrating how the framework may be utilised. Within this discussion, elements of disaster planning and response that fall within each of the three domains have been identified as follows: human capacity (HC); social ecology (SE); and culture and values (CV).

Modifications to the PWG framework: disrupted resources

Disrupted resource 1: physical well-being

In any disaster situation, the immediate priority is to remove casualties and bystanders to a place of safety (HC). This requires some planning to ensure there is a sufficient and efficient number of professionals and volunteers trained to respond effectively and administer triaging and transportation of victims to hospitals and morgues. The physical integrity of the area needs to be safeguarded prior to any first responder entering the area. In some instances specialist engineers and equipment may be required to ensure the area is structurally safe. The equipment

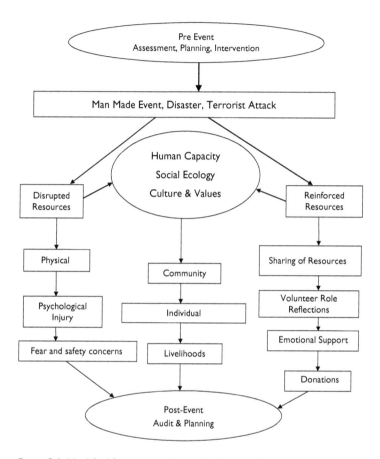

Figure 8.1 Modified framework for use in disaster planning

necessary to carry out the recovery work should be available, along with sufficient vehicles and open roadways to transport the casualties to hospitals or places of safety.

Once these priorities are met, the immediate basic needs of survivors in mass disaster situations will be food, safety, shelter and financial support. These needs can be met partly through the community support by the sharing of resources such as food, water and shelter (SE), as occurred in Bali. In large-scale disasters, further food and emergency provisions and supplies will need to be provided to ensure the maintenance of emergency supplies at outreach posts. Emergency supplies of food need to be dropped off to seriously ill, disabled, vulnerable and elderly members of the community. In addition, in a large-scale disaster situation, temporary housing, clean water and sanitation will need to be provided – all basic necessities required for the physical needs (HC) of the affected population.

Disrupted resource 2: psychological well-being

Following a catastrophic event, psychosocial symptoms (HC) will be evident in most survivors, their families, some community members and first responders. Rather than rush into 'mental health diagnosis', health care workers, mental health professionals and those in support roles need to be trained (HC) to adopt a minimalist 'watch and wait approach', and be encouraged to initially use a basic empathetic and supportive approach with the victims. Priority must be given to reuniting people to their families, friends and communities (SE), as it is here that the victims are most likely to receive the emotional support they require, as evidenced by the study participants in both Bali and Perth and the literature.

A specialised trained group of volunteers will be required to co-ordinate this reunification with family members. Health professionals, family members and victims will need to be provided with information to enable them to recognise prolonged symptoms of mental health difficulties, particularly after the first month. The Australian Red Cross have produced an information booklet for victims and families in a major crisis (Valent *et al*, 2008). Those victims experiencing ongoing symptoms will require referral to an appropriate mental health professional.

Disrupted resource 3: family livelihoods

At the individual and family levels there will be disruption to economic resources (HC). Victims may be unable to work due to personal injury or because their job no longer exists as a direct consequence of the disaster, such as destruction of the place of employment or economic fallout (as occurred in Bali). Families lose the economic provision of victims who were killed or injured, and the economy and businesses are depleted of victims' skills input. Local and federal governments therefore need to include adequate financial provision for families and training of existing workers to help replace the skills of workers who have been lost or injured, particularly in essential industries such as water, electricity, transport and oil and gas supply. In a large-scale disaster or terrorist attack they may also need to provide for downturns in the economy, such as occurred in Bali when tourists stopped arriving.

Disrupted resource 4: fear and safety concerns

Post-event the victims and many community members will fear for their safety, as well as the safety of their family members (CV). Effective decision-making and appraisal of their own and others' safety is often compromised by their involvement in the disaster. Links and announcements to reassure individuals, families and communities, in addition to information regarding support, could be provided through churches, newspapers, television, newsletters, community radio announcements, the internet, phone, tweets and texts. Reporting of continuing investigations and efforts to catch the perpetrators will also help to allay the fears of the population.

Reinforced resources

Reinforced resources 1: sharing of resources

The immediate period following a disaster sees a 'wave of compassion, goodwill and care' and community outpouring of assistance (Rao, 2006, p. 502). Offers of food, medicine, shelter and monetary donations and promises of help abound. In Bali and Perth the local communities rallied around with food, monetary donations and emotional support. Many participants in this study described the benefits they felt from the practical and emotional support of family, friends and neighbours. This widespread sharing of resources is a prime example of the social connectedness involved in community and collective responses to the disruption and impact caused by a disaster (SE). Effective collation, co-ordination and distribution of donations is an important consideration for response agencies. In Bali this was one of the areas where volunteers reported stress and tension, as large quantities of donations had to be stored, catalogued and distributed and looting and theft had to be prevented.

Reinforced resources 2: volunteering

It is also recognised that disasters or complex emergencies can have beneficial effects, such as people feeling motivated to altruistic actions (HC). As a result of the motivation to assist and help in any way, it is not unusual to see many local people who live near a disaster scene arrive at the scene first, to take on the role of first responders to an attack (Bisson and Cohen, 2006). Hence, it is recommended that community training courses, particularly in basic first aid, be available to community members to ensure that responders can administer first aid in a safe and efficient manner, in an effort to minimise loss of life. In cases where there is a large influx of volunteers, there will be a need to take charge of organisation and allocation of tasks appropriate to volunteers' skill levels. Hence rostering, pre-registration and training of a disaster emergency response corps would be beneficial.

Reinforced resources 3: emotional support

Victims turn to family and friends as soon as possible in the aftermath of a disaster. Victims in Bali and Perth reported the emotional support of family and friends as a crucial element of their recovery. This 'social bonding' is considered a form of 'unity against a common enemy' – namely, the perpetrators (Strang and Ager, 2001, p. 4). As a result of the stress of providing emotional support, family members and friends can become secondary victims. As a preventative measure they should be provided detailed, practical and easy-to-read information from mental health and relief agencies which encourages self-care, as well as tips on how to support family members in crisis.

Reinforced resources 4: donations

As well as local communities sharing food, shelter and monetary donations, national and international communities will donate medicines, personnel, tents, food and clothing. In Perth the monetary donations to the Red Cross after the Bali bombing alone amounted to A$15.3 million (Australian Red Cross, 2005). Medicine donations from the local and international community were over-whelming. Most medicine donations were extremely useful, although a few were not as they were out of date, labelled in a language other than Indonesian or inappropriate for the immediate needs of the victims (World Health Organiza-tion, 2003). The management, logistics and legalities surrounding storage and timely distribution of donations – especially vital medical aid – is an important consideration for planning organisations.

Post-event: assessment, evaluation and planning

This modified framework was developed as a result of the study carried out after the Bali disaster in 2002. Its recommendations are based on comprehensive anal-ysis of the participants' experiences and recommendations in Bali and Perth. The rationale behind the framework is that in any large-scale disaster, existing organ-isations are often overwhelmed by the tragedy with which they are faced and need all the support that is offered. The first step is to form a task force consisting of community members, ambulance and police officials, community organisa-tions, volunteers and engineers. Their task will be to form a comprehensive psy-chosocial approach to disaster response in their area. The modified framework presented in Figure 8.1 and the subsequent discussion provides some guidelines on how the framework may be used. It is recognised that each disaster has its own set of locally specific demands. It is essential to work methodically and assess the existing local resources. Where there are potential deficiencies, it is impor-tant that sufficient resources are provided to build resources to a level that will meet the stresses and demands raised by a disaster. If used appropriately, the framework enhances the chances of an efficient and culturally appropriate response.

Post-disaster

The PWG framework provides an opportunity to assess and evaluate the effective-ness of disaster responses. As survivors and their relatives have essential insights into disaster response, they should be invited to participate in post-disaster assess-ment teams. The team should also include those people and organisations that formed the initial planning team. Information from key stakeholders in the response is essential; such stakeholders should include police, ambulance officers, the fire brigade, community organisations, victims and family members. Reports and information from interviews and focus groups should form part of the audit. The key purpose of the team would be to audit the response to the disaster, as well as formulating a new strategic plan for emergency response should another disaster occur.

The framework and domains could be a starting point to assess the type of resources that were depleted and reinforced during the disaster. The audit could reveal ways in which the planning team could build and replenish these resources. Further examples of strategies to enhance planning and response are contained in the next section, which presents the recommendations arising from the study.

Recommendations for future disaster management

It is imperative in any crisis situation that disaster intervention must take into account the setting, culture and context. Included in each recommendation is information which explains some background to the recommendations. It is not intended for the recommendations to take the place of a detailed emergency management plan. The aim is for the recommendations to be considered by the organisations or individuals that undertake such work and to encourage them, if they are not already doing so, to take a psychosocial approach to their work.[1]

Recommendations for immediate assistance

- Priority to be given to injured who require efficient and timely triaging. In Bali this was not undertaken well, and it is likely this resulted in a number of casualties (World Health Organization, 2003) that may have been prevented had the bystanders who were first on the scene been trained in disaster first aid. In the immediate post-event stage the next priority is for provision of food, safety, water, shelter and support that enables the reunification of surviving victims with their family and friends.
- Professional mental health workers and response personnel need to take a 'watch and wait' approach with victims of the disaster, as most individuals will recover from their symptoms over a period of time. In most cases it is likely to be clinically unwise to make a diagnosis within the first month post-event as this will be too early to distinguish a victim's trauma symptoms.
- It is important that all emergency responders are aware of the range of responses that can be considered normal reactions to very abnormal circumstances, and be ready to give the basic levels of emotional and practical support required.
- Administration of questionnaires or supportive interviews may be required to identify those at risk within these groups, with targeted interventions and specialised referral instigated where necessary (Valent et al, 2008; Bisson, 2007).

Recommendations for training and disaster response

- There needs to be provision of specific disaster first aid courses for interested members of the general public and community organisations. This could occur under the usual first aid training organisations such as St John's Ambulance.
- Volunteers and professionals need to be taught the importance of self-regulation so that they operate within their own safety skill levels.
- Training of professional responders such as the police, ambulance drivers and local volunteers to include disaster first aid, fire-fighting, psychological first aid and personal and victim safety considerations is paramount.
- The use of self-help leaflets, newspaper and television advertising can help in the post-disaster stage. These may facilitate identification of those victims who require further assistance and aid their progress to the next phase of specialised assessment and support from mental or other professional health providers.
- The basics of self-care, such as regular breaks, regular fluid and food intake and identifying signs of undue psychological and physical distress, need to be emphasised in any specialised first response training.
- A response team trained to give practical support as well as psychological first aid should be made available for the duration of the emergency, as well as post-event, to monitor the response team. Personnel who show significant signs of distress should be temporarily removed from the situation.
- Training for professional and volunteer responders regarding the need to be respectful of each other and each other's knowledge is essential.

Recommendations for government

- A joint committee of government and non-government agencies and local volunteer responders should be formed which meets regularly to formulate a response plan. It is recommended that this be established in any major city that may be vulnerable to a terrorist attack or major complex emergencies or disasters.
- The local community needs to be included in any future planning, as community members are often first on the scene, be it a terrorist attack, natural disaster, train derailment or fire. As Shover states: 'each disaster response begins with the individual's preparedness at the local level and all disaster preparedness must incorporate training of health professionals, citizens and families in disaster drills' (Shover, 2007, p. 4).
- A task force can be formed with the prime aim of calling for volunteers willing to help in, for example, an Australian-based volunteer force of emergency responders. While NGOs such as the Red Cross have a roster of emergency volunteers, they are unlikely to have sufficient personnel to be available to help in a mass casualty situation.

- A call for general as well as specific volunteers would be helpful. This would be a similar concept to that announced by Kevin Rudd, Australia's Prime Minister during the Bali bombing, of an overseas civilian corps of 500 volunteers willing to help in disaster-affected areas overseas (*The Australian*, 2009). The specific community members required might include nurses, doctors, psychologists, engineers, plumbers, electricians, builders, fire-fighters and ambulance drivers. General volunteers would consist of locals and may include those willing to dig or search for survivors, such as occurred in the recent earthquake disaster in Haiti, or those willing to take charge of telephone enquiries or provide food for the responders.

Recommendations for policy and practice

- Information leaflets to be produced to help family members and friends support their family member who is injured or distressed. A 'hint list' and 'what to do if. . .' tips based around the principles of psychological first aid can be included. A similar form was issued during the Bali disaster, although helplines and volunteer counsellors and professional organisations still received a high level of calls from concerned relatives.
- Sufficient helplines need to be operational as soon as possible after the disaster as a source of information for all who may require it, as well as a referral base if callers need to be assessed by mental health professionals.
- Co-ordination and registration of volunteers is essential. The responsibility for this could be undertaken by a specially formed organisation consisting of members of other emergency response organisations such as the Red Cross, St John's Ambulance, the police, church and community organisations.
- Collation of volunteer contact details makes co-ordination and recruitment of volunteers to the scene easier in the initial stages. An electronic and written register of names, addresses and telephone numbers is crucial.
- Educational material and training should be given to emergency response personnel to enable them to self-monitor for signs of undue distress, and particularly for signs of excessive fatigue. A confidential helpline should be set up to enable volunteers and professional responders to call for emotional support during and after the event.
- If the response is prolonged, some downtime for volunteers and professional responders is essential. In the initial busy stages of a response just a few moments of downtime away from the site would be useful if possible, as first responders tend to override the signs of their own physical and psychological exhaustion. This was evident during the response to the Bali attack by both volunteers and professional responders, in Bali and in Perth.
- The provision of simple recreational activities is a useful consideration if the response continues for several weeks. A number of the volunteers in Bali mentioned the usefulness of basic recreational activities in helping them relax and de-stress.

- An information pack including leaflets regarding psychological first aid should be produced by all authorities involved in pre-planning a disaster response, and community organisations could be issued with a stockpile of information packs before any disaster.
- Due to variations in the media's conduct during the aftermath of an attack, the code of conduct for all media should be reviewed and mandated.

All of the above recommendations need to be funded by government budgets and emergency contingency funding to provide for disaster planning.

Limitations

There are always limitations or caveats that need to be acknowledged when undertaking research. There are inherent difficulties in conducting fieldwork in any country. Issues of difference of language, culture and custom all have to be considered. Concepts of 'time' and 'quality' are all culture-bound and the reliance on local knowledge from treasured research assistants in Bali was not just paramount in the success of our data collection, but imperative to the entire Bali study. However, it has to be acknowledged that meaning can be lost as a result of the bi-directional nature of communication needed to carry out this research endeavour. There is also a great difficulty in finding participants who are willing to discuss and essentially 're-live' parts of what was and still is a traumatic and unpleasant time of their life and the histories of Bali and the Kingsley Football Club in Perth. The research process is one that ultimately requires the vast amount of data collected to be analysed and interpreted in a way that honours the stories of the individuals, but also inevitably to some extent aggregates the messages in the data. This enables authors to present a rich and meaningful depiction of the 'voices' of the participants, and has been done in this case with respect to the information and the research process.

Significance and implications of the study

For policy and advocacy and funding

A terrorist attack challenges the individual and the community in many ways, and it is clear there is much more work to be done and a need for increased research funding in this all-important area. Bushfire disasters are increasing in Australia, and Australian Research Council-funded research now aims at understanding the long-term disaster needs for individuals affected by the Black Saturday bushfires (Melbourne Sustainable Society Institute, 2010). The distress endured by victims and family members after terrorist attacks, the reactions reported by first responders to undertaking their roles and responsibilities and the conflicts that interfere with the efficiency of the volunteer response are worthy of further consideration and funding.

Local residents require training in disaster first aid and disaster response, as they are usually the first to respond to a terrorist attack. Such training will equip them with the necessary skills to enable them to give the best support possible in a disaster response and to help reduce the loss of life. It is training that will also be invaluable in other situations requiring first aid in which they may become involved. While Australia has not been a target of a large-scale terrorist attack, it is important the government does not become complacent. For example, in 2010 the Australian government announced input of A$1.1 billion to enhance Australia's protection capabilities in Afghanistan (Faulkner, 2010, p. 1).

It is also proposed that targeted funding is required to support the training of local volunteers, mental health experts and police, fire and ambulance personnel in preparation for a disaster response. Family and friends have been shown to be the main source of emotional support for victims of terrorist attacks. Sufficient funding is required to undertake essential research and disseminate information that enables them to effectively carry out this important task. Such research could also inform the production and dissemination of information to help those in this support role. This could be disseminated, for example, online, in print, on the radio and through social media.

While not all victims of a disaster will require the services of a mental health professional, those who do will need a professional who is trained and equipped with specialised skills. All who respond to help in a terrorist attack can experience compassion fatigue, burnout and vicarious trauma. The effects can be severe and long-lasting. Free specialised mental health support must be available to all responders in the initial and subsequent stages of a disaster. Government funds are required to provide subsidised training for health professionals interested in training in post-disaster medicine and counselling. Teaching and training schools in university departments of medicine, psychology and sociology may need to extend the postgraduate courses they provide to include specialised courses in disaster response and supporting terrorist victims.

For psychologists and counsellors

This study has highlighted that not all victims of terrorist attacks require professional mental health support. Instead of responding immediately with a pathology focus, psychologists need to adopt a 'watch and wait' approach for at least one month, as until then most victims will be exhibiting normal distress reactions. The term 'compassionate witnessing' explains the focus of this gentle supportive approach (Weingarten, 2006, p. 16). In a large-scale disaster, psychological services will be overwhelmed; it is therefore important that community members, voluntary groups and other first-line agency personnel be trained in psychological first aid. Psychologists will need to work collaboratively with these personnel. To enhance their effectiveness in large-scale disaster response, psychologists will need specialised training to equip them with the knowledge to respond in these complex situations. During their response to a disaster, psychologists will urgently need to assess and prioritise the many victims that seek help and seek peer supervision and emotional support, to help ensure they do not also become victims.

For future research

Terrorist attacks kill, injure and induce fear in many countries across the world. Research which centres on the subject of terrorist attacks, especially in developing countries has increased in the past decade. Terrorist attacks have multiple layers of effects and require multiple layers of support. Further research is required surrounding the resources and resilience that pre-exist in communities and how they can be mobilised in the event of a large-scale terrorist attack or disaster.

When attacks occur, many bystanders and volunteers rush to help. Research which examines how we can best equip first responders to reduce the loss of life that occurs in such attacks is an urgent necessity. As we have seen in Bali, in Perth and in the recent bushfire response in Australia, too often there is a lack of leadership and confusion, particularly in terms of who takes charge of the situation (Teague *et al*, 2009). Planning and joint co-ordination is key to an orderly response to any form of disaster and is worthy of further study. Finally, there is a need for research which examines the effects and types of support required for those who endure a disproportionate amount of the disaster burden, such as women, children, the sick, those with a mental illness and those from low socio-economic backgrounds.

Conclusion

While the best way of dealing with terrorist attacks is to prevent them from occurring in the first place, history indicates to us that we have not yet been successful in this endeavour. For these individuals and communities involved, such attacks were and remain life-altering events. However long the world waits until the next terrorist attack, we will continue to see and hear the impact of these events in all forms of social media, as well as driving the government to debate and respond to the challenges that were brought about by the attacks. It is important to remember, however, that while these terrorist attacks are all-encompassing events for individuals at the time they occur, they form part of the history of the communities who eventually demonstrate resilience at a societal level.

Since 9/11, the Bali and Mumbai attacks, the London bombing and the Asian tsunami a resurgence of research interest in the area of post-disaster support has taken place. As this book goes to press conflicts have escalated in Syria and Iraq, causing untold human displacement, terror and killings. As the book goes to press, the US government has declared military action against ISIL, and the Prime Minister of Australia, Hon Tony Abbott MP, has committed troops and military support. September 2014 has been in many ways a difficult month with the beheading of several journalists and aid workers, and thousands of civilians fleeing Iraq, Kurdistan and Syria. Research and advocacy does not seem sufficient, and there is a sense that there is much more knowledge to be uncovered regarding what causes these attacks in the first place, what action governments should take to prevent them and the effects and types of support which best suit the needs of the many levels of victims.

However long the world waits until the next terrorist attack, we will continue to see and hear the impact of these events in all forms of social media. Governments will continue to be driven to debate and will respond to the challenges that were brought about by the attacks. This book and the study it was based around have attempted to add to the body of knowledge of this subject. The participants' experiences, information from the literature, the researchers' observations and official reports post attack have all been an invaluable source of information. To enhance the efficacy of response it is suggested that existing community resources need to be utilised, local volunteers and professional volunteers need to be recruited and trained in disaster response and lessons need to be learnt from other terrorist attacks. In doing so it is likely the efficacy of response will be enhanced, more lives will be saved and all victims will be given the level of support they richly deserve.

Note

1 Where aspects of the recommendations were previously utilised in Bali or Perth, due acknowledgement is made. Where this occurs there is a tacit recommendation for improvement in these areas.

References

The Australian (2009, 25 October). Civilian corps to compliment assistance: Kevin Rudd. Retrieved 20 Aug 2014 from http://www.theaustralian.com.au/news/nation/civilian-corps-to-complement-assistance-kevin-rudd/story-e6frg6nf-225791031127

Australian Red Cross (2005). *Bali Assistance Program – Australia Appeal.* Retrieved 20 Aug 2014 from http://www.redcross.org.au/ourservices_aroundtheworld_emergency relief_bali_assistanceprogram.htm

Bisson, J. I. (2007). Post traumatic stress disorder. *Occupational Medicine, 57*(6), 399–403. Retrieved 20 Aug 2014 from http://occmed.oxfordjournals.org/content/57/6/399.full

Bisson, J. I., and Cohen, J. A. (2006). Disseminating early interventions following trauma. *Journal of Traumatic Stress, 19*(5), 583–595.

El Haq, E. (2007). Community reponse to climatic hazards in Northern Pakistan. *Mountain Research and Development, 27*(4), 308–312. doi:10.1659/mrd.0947

Faulkner, J. (2010). *Budget 2010–1: Defence budget overview.* Retrieved 20 Aug 2014 from http://www.defence.gov.au/minister/Faulknertpl.cfm?CurrentId=10273

Fjord, L., and Manderson, L. (2009). Anthropological perspectives on disasters and disability: An introduction. *Human Organization, 68*(1), 64–72. Retrieved 20 Aug 2014 from http://search.proquest.com/docview/201171341?accountid=10382

Hollis, M. (2007). *Formulating disaster recovery plans for New Zealand: using a case study of the 1931 Napier earthquake.* (Master's thesis). Retrieved 20 Aug 2014 from http://ir.canterbury.ac.nz/bitstream/10092/1456/1/thesis_fulltext.pdf

Inter-Agency Standing Committee (IASC) 4th Working Draft (2006). *Guidance on mental health and psychosocial support in emergency settings*. Inter-Agency Standing Committee, 4–80. Retrieved 20 Aug 2014 from http://www.who.int/mental_health/emergencies/guidelinesiasc_mental_health_psychosocial_june_2007.pdf

Larson, R. C., Metzger, M. D., and Cahn, M. F. (2006). Responding to emergencies: Lessons learned and the need for analysis. *Interfaces, 36*(96), 486–501.

Melbourne Sustainable Society Institute. (2010). *ARC Linkage Grant: Bushfires, social connectedness and mental health*. Retrieved 20 Aug 2014 from http://sustainable.unimelb.edu.au/content/pages/arc-linkage-grant-bushfires-social-connectedness-and-mental-health

Moscardino, U., Scrimin, S., Capello, F., and Altoe, G. (2010). Social support, sense of community, collective values, and depressive symptoms in adolescent survivors of the 2004 Beslan terrorist attack. *Social Science and Medicine, 70*, 27–34.

Psychosocial Working Group (PWG) (2003). *Psychosocial intervention in complex emergencies: A framework for practice*. Working Paper, Centre for International Health Studies, Queen Margaret University, Edinburgh.

Rao, K. (2006). Psychosocial support in disaster-affected communities. *International Review of Psychiatry, 18*(6), 501–505. doi:1237467351

Shover, H. (2007). Understanding the chain of communication during a disaster. *Perspective in Psychiatric Care, 43*(1), 4–14.

Steury, S., Spencer, S., and Parkinson, G. W. (2004). The social context of recovery. *Psychiatry: Interpersonal and Biological Processes, 67*(2), 158–163.

Strang, A. B., and Ager, A. (2001). *Building a conceptual framework for psychosocial intervention in complex emergencies: Reporting on the work of the Psychosocial Working Group*, 1–6. Centre for International Health Studies, Queen Margaret University, Edinburgh.

Teague, B., McLeod, R., and Pascoe, S. (2009). *The 2009 Victorian Bushfires Royal Commission final report*. Retrieved 20 Aug 2014 from http://www.apo.org.au/research/2009-victorian-bushfires-royal-commission-final-report

Trappler, B. (2010, 31 August). Post traumatic stress: Symptoms, diagnosis and brain mechanisms. *Psychology Today*, 1–4.

Valent, P., Berah, E., Jones, J., Wrath, R., and Hill, J. (2008). *Coping with a major personal crisis: Emergency REDi Plan*. Retrieved 20 Aug 2014 from http://www.redcross.org.au/ourservices_acrossaustralia_disasteremergencyservices_recover_coping.htm

Vijaykumar, L., Thara, R., John, S., and Chellappa, S. (2006). Psychosocial intervention after tsunami in Tamil Nadu, India. *International Review of Psychiatry, 18*(3), 225–231.

Weingarten, K. (2006). *Compassionate witnessing and the transformation of societal violence: How individuals can make a difference*, 1–21. Retrieved 20 Aug 2014 from http://www.witnessingproject.org/articles/CompassionateWitnessing.pdf

World Health Organization (2003). *Workshop on disaster management for the health sector in Indonesia: Lessons learned from the Bali bomb*. Bali, Indonesia.

A reflective diary and photograph narratives

By Gwen Brookes

Dance as if no one were watching, sing as if no one were listening and live each day as if it were your last.

(Anonymous Irish saying)

This book started life as a research project that evolved with the first author's response to a terrorist attack in Bali in 2002, when seven members of the local football team in Perth were killed and many more injured. A total of 88 Australians died in the attack, which claimed the lives of a total of 202 people and injured more than 200. In response, Gwen, the first author – a psychologist – volunteered, along with many others, to act as a support to the club, the players and the families of the injured and bereaved. It was a privileged position and she thought, like many of the victims and family members, that some good should come out of something so sad and brutal.

That privilege was extended when she was granted permission to interview 50 victims of the disaster in Bali and Perth and the PhD research project outlined in this book commenced. Co-authors of the book, Jaya Earnest and Julie Ann Pooley, were invaluable sources of support and wisdom throughout the project and were Gwen's supervisors throughout its production. They were a natural choice to be part of the team producing this book.

On 12 October 2012, hundreds of survivors, their families and friends and those who had lost loved ones in the attack travelled to Bali to attend a ceremony to mark the tenth anniversary of the bombing. It was memorable in many ways for everyone, including the first author, who felt privileged to travel with a group of people from the Kingsley Football Club which she had supported and had remained in contact with following the disaster in 2002. It was a difficult time for all, as a number of the returning victims and family members were journeying to Bali for the first time since the bombing. There were press reports that they too were going to be targets of a terrorist attack on the island, and it was rumoured that threats had been made.

The Indonesian government took the threats very seriously and armed protection was provided for everyone on the trip, especially on the journey to and from the memorial service. Some 2,000 military and police officers, including snipers, were deployed to protect the civilians and dignitaries. Armed guards

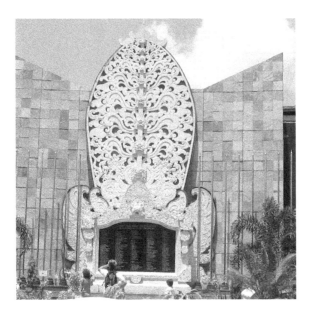

Photograph 1 Bali memorial

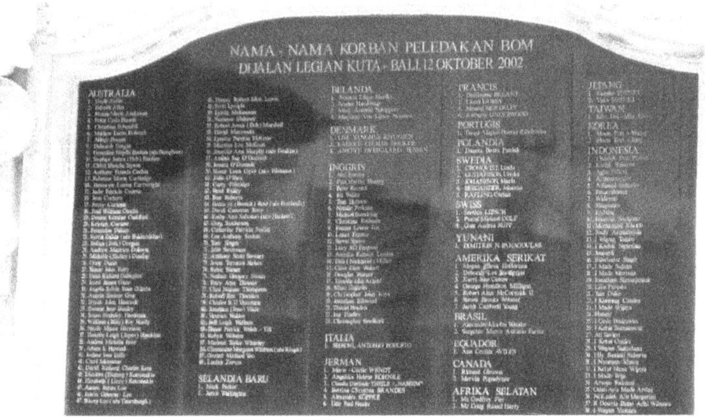

Photograph 2 List of names of those who lost their lives

with machine guns were positioned inside the buses which transported the attendees to the ceremony and armed motorbike riders were positioned at the front and rear of each bus in a long convoy of vehicles heading to the ceremony. Yet the place it was held – a disused quarry within the Garuda Wisnu Kencana Cultural Park, high above Kuta – was a peaceful and fitting setting for the many dignitaries and relatives of those who had been killed or injured to make their speeches. In a poignant part of the service, the names of all who had lost their lives were read out.

It was a hot and humid day, with the intense Balinese sun beating down on all who attended. Volunteers passed bottles of water along the many lines of people from across the world who had gathered to remember those that had lost their lives. It was a moving and dignified service to mark the tenth anniversary. Carefully chosen music formed a background to the proceedings as well as a remembrance wall of photographs of those who had lost their lives. For once, the media seemed to keep a dignified distance to allow those attending to grieve and to remember. Many sobs of sadness echoed throughout the quarry, yet for many it was almost the end of a journey, with some closure. At the end of the service people queued to quietly await their turn to place a small floral tribute in the remembrance pool. In the many services held throughout the countries touched by the disaster, no one would forget what had happened, but many would report a shift in their emotions to one of quiet acceptance of what had happened.

Reflective photo-narrative commentary

The photographs in this section were taken during my field trip to Bali. It is intended in this set of photographs to capture the essence of Bali beyond the usual tourist venues and to visually represent the difficult socio-economic circumstances endured on a daily basis by a large proportion of the population – circumstances made even more difficult by the Bali bombings of 2002 and the subsequent economic downturn. Many of us holiday there frequently and love Bali; it is also important to remember that its inhabitants are extremely proud and resilient.

Two months after the bombing a women's sewing co-operative, 'Adopt a Co-Op', was set up by an Australian couple to enable five widows with ten children between them to set up a business making t-shirts, polo shirts and bags for hotels, tourists, sports groups and schools. The photographs below illustrate their workshop, their

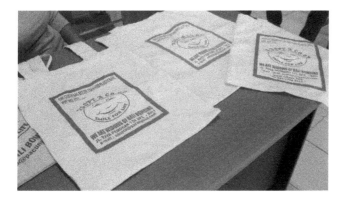

Photograph 3 Bags sewn by the Women's Sewing Co-operative

equipment and some of the members. I went there on a number of occasions to interview participants and to purchase some t-shirts to bring back home. I couldn't help noticing how cramped the conditions were and how ancient some of the sewing machines appeared. Yet the goods produced were of a very high standard and the women were always smiling and laughing, with noisy chatter rising above the busy sounds of the machines at every visit. The income from the business is modest but vitally important, as it helps the women to earn an income to support their families and to maintain a sense of pride and independence. The co-operative is also a place for mutual understanding and support when needed.

Research assistants

The photograph below portrays Sherley hard at work translating the interviews and Chakra with me on one of our many field trips. Sherley and Chakra were two

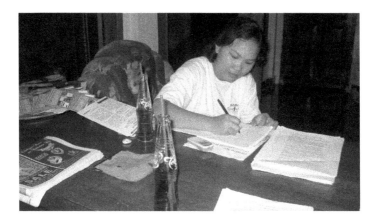

Photograph 4 Research assistant Sherly

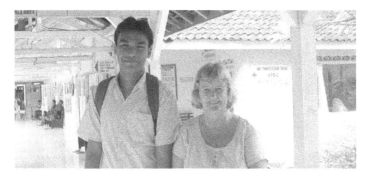

Photograph 5 Research assistant Cakra and Gwen Brookes at Denpasar hospital

of the workers seconded from YKIDS to be my research assistants. Shirley and Chakra were invaluable sources of information regarding cultural norms in Bali, as well as efficient and cheerful companions who remain my friends today. The bottles of cool cold tea visible are generally what the lovely participants bought us on site visits.

A snapshot of the socio-cultural milieu

The interviews I undertook in Bali had a significant impact on a personal and emotional level, almost on a daily basis. The stories were always sad and emotional. I do not want to give the impression that the Bali stories were vastly different or less tragic than the Perth stories. It is just the Bali stories were, from a socio-economic perspective, so very different, for many reasons. As I was immersed in data collection in Bali for two months I could see and experience the very poor socio-economic circumstances most participants had to endure. I could walk out of my hotel behind the shops and restaurants and see the housing conditions of the hotel workers and other victims who had experienced the bombing at close quarters. They lived well below the poverty line in sparse and usually overcrowded houses.

As a result there was more to the stories in Bali than the obvious grief that abounded, and this section will reveal a little of that for the reader. This time the stories contain my personal reflections and are based on my daily notes and personal reflections. The following is an overview of just one day of interview and data collection in Bali. I wrote the stories in narrative form because it hopefully gives an insight into the socio-cultural milieu the interviews were conducted in. They are also a snapshot into my emotional journey in Bali, and catalogue a few of the real-life situations I experienced in my role as a researcher.

The fifth day

I remember the fifth day of the interviews as being particularly draining both physically and psychologically. It was a very hot, humid and energy-sapping day. I hadn't slept well and we were having trouble locating a number of people and their houses. The driver was unable to negotiate the narrow streets which lead to the housing compounds by car. As a result we all had to walk a few blocks each time, in the hot, humid conditions. My hair was often stuck to my face with sweat and my face was glowing red with the heat. I must have looked quite amusing to all, as I was dressed in long sleeves, long pants, socks and closed shoes in an effort to protect myself from the mosquitoes which buzzed around during the daytime and at dusk.

This was the third interview of the fifth day. We were in a poor inner-city area of Denpasar. It was pouring with rain and the occasional clap of thunder and noisy dogs seemed to add to the drama of the day. The drains were overflowing and large pools of stagnant water were everywhere. It was lapping at the front steps of some of the houses, and the smell of dampness and stagnant water was everywhere. There were a number of thin and hungry-looking dogs wandering up and down the road. All of the houses, of which there were about six, were built of hardboard and a tin roof.

We were searching for the first address and a young woman stopped to ask in English whether we were the people who wanted to talk to the Bali victims. We said we were and she said she had been injured in the bombing and eagerly offered to be interviewed. As she fitted the interview criteria I agreed to her being interviewed, as she seemed very keen to talk to us. This unexpected participant followed us to Jayu's house and told her she was going to be interviewed there too. When I queried this from the privacy point of view, the doctor and everyone else smiled and reassured me that this was fine. By the end of the interview I realised that there seemed to be an open-door policy in this participant's house, as a number of people arrived unannounced throughout the interview to listen to what we were doing for a while and then would leave with as little announcement as they had arrived with. I thought they were relatives of Jayu's, but when I queried, I was told they were friends and neighbours who were curious and just wanted to listen for a bit. I quickly realised that privacy as we know it in the west was not an issue.

It just seemed natural for us all to pile into the one house to conduct the interviews. There were two rooms in the house. It was typical of most of the houses in Denpasar, in that one room was for cooking, watching television and socialising in and the other for sleeping in. The conditions were cramped and sparse. There was little decoration except for a few pictures on the wall, and little furniture except for a table with colourful plastic flowers on and a small lounge suite with a few low cane chairs on one side of the room. Yet it was a home – a lovely home at that, with a beautiful atmosphere of peace and a welcoming air. By the standards of Balinese houses it was larger than usual and had more furniture than the other houses I had visited that day: the furniture in those houses consisted of a mattress on the floor, two plastic stools and a small table, with a small cooking stove in the corner.

During the interview Jayu's 7-year-old son fell asleep across her lap. So we had two participants, myself and the research assistant, two neighbours and the interviewee's son all crowded into a small house to conduct the interviews. This didn't seem ideal, and constantly plucked at my psychologist and researcher's notion of the importance of privacy at all times. As it didn't seem to be bothering the interviewees we continued the interviews one at a time. As we commenced one interview, yet another neighbour joined us and brought jack fruit and bread for us all to eat. It was becoming quite a social occasion and I had to relax and just go with the moment, with what was happening.

Before we commenced, drinks were purchased for myself and the research assistant from the outside shop. I couldn't refuse, and neither could I pay for the drinks. My interpreter was quite firm on this and, when I quietly offered, told me it would be deemed disrespectful. Yet I knew this participant could not afford them. It was not unusual for this to happen: it is an important part of the warm Balinese culture of hospitality to look after guests by offering them soft drinks and sometimes food.

The two interviews took quite a long time, as everyone often broke into lively chat about the bombing or other, often non-related, topics. It was hard to ignore the street activities going on outside: the noisy barking dogs, people on motorbikes driving around the neighbourhood, children happily playing in the street and the street seller selling food and other goods, announcing his arrival by ringing a bell. I felt privileged to be given an insight into the Bali far removed from the glitzy hotels in which many tourists would stay. I felt guilty to be returning to my very comfortable hotel room, which was probably similar in size to the home in which this participant was living with four of her family.

The interviews continue

The next interview of the day was in an even poorer part of the city. There were four houses placed in a square, although in reality each consisted of one room. I sat on a bench outside, as the woman of the house said this was best. I got the feeling she didn't want me to go inside. I didn't mean to peek but, when one of the curtains was moved to allow someone to come outside, I could see a mattress on the floor, and that it was very dark inside. All around me were pigeons hanging in cages, chickens roaming freely and large birds in cages; an angry-looking dog was chained to the ground just a few metres away from us. In total there were four rooms, with about ten people living in close proximity to each other. There were no doors, just curtains across each opening, and no windows that I could see.

The next participant was a middle-aged woman and although we couldn't speak each other's language, we were still able to communicate. It was almost as

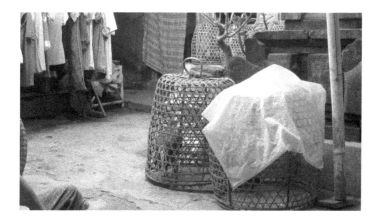

Photograph 6 A family courtyard

if we had a spiritual and emotional connection. Again the family sent out for drinks for me which I knew they could not afford. It seemed a noisy, dusty and difficult environment in which to conduct an interview and I wondered how people survived in such an environment. There was a young girl who was about 12 months old in a baby stroller darting in and out, skilfully avoiding the chickens who roamed freely in the small courtyard. The baby had a bad cold and chesty cough and a constantly streaming nose. I couldn't help thinking the conditions in which she was living would not have helped. Yet the families seemed happy, the children were well cared for and the interview was filled with much laughter.

The last interview of the day was conducted in the back streets of Sanur, some miles from Kuta. The village was completely flooded so that water lapped up to the front step of the houses. There were large ponds of stagnant water everywhere. In the house in which I conducted the interview, the children were sick with tuberculosis. I felt sorry for this participant as I knew she had financial difficulties which compounded her problems. Once I learned the children were at school and were on medication for TB I felt quite relieved, as they were at least getting the treatment they needed. Unkempt, sick dogs roamed up and down the street. There were clouds of mosquitoes hovering over the pools of water and in dark corners of the house. I felt physically very uncomfortable and emotionally very sad that the people were so poor and had no choice but to live in these conditions.

Time and time again, at each interview, the dire economic plight of the participants and the need for more money, food and employment would be raised. This participant's plight seemed much worse than that of any of the other interviewees that day. She was a widow struggling to bring up her two sick children in very poor conditions. The poverty this family endured is difficult to describe, and writing about it does not really capture their plight. She was trying to make a living by taking in sewing and selling some basic items at the front of her house.

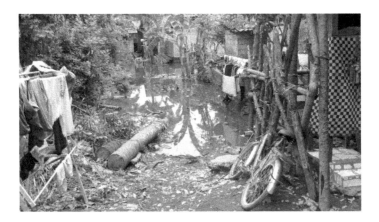

Photograph 7 The flooded paths

There weren't more than a dozen items for sale, such as soap, razors and sachets of washing powder.

I had to hold back the tears at this interview. Suffice to say they were one of the poorest families I have ever met. A baby kitten was at the front entrance to the house, and it was clearly sick and dying. My driver seemed to sense my extreme sadness as we left the house. What he said to me almost seemed to sum up the day: 'life goes on, yesterday is yesterday, today is today and tomorrow is tomorrow'. I think this was the Balinese equivalent of 'tomorrow is another day'. I couldn't help but think that the sadness was all my sadness, as most of the people seemed to have accepted their situation. There really wasn't any other option.

Summary

The areas I visited that day seemed even more economically depressed than any I had ever visited in my many travels around the world. I have never seen such poverty and I felt pangs of guilt at having so much. I wanted to empty my purse and give the families whatever money I had. My rescuing mode was in full swing and yet ethically, deep down, I knew it was not something I could or should do. The descriptions I have given are an insight into life in Bali beyond the tourist hotels and beaches. It is a picture of life that maybe we in the west should envy, as in many ways they are not sad stories per se; they are stories of hope, resilience and determination, all of which the participants demonstrated in abundance. I saw communities that share and care, and where kinship and friendship abounded. They welcomed me into their hearts and their homes just like the people we interviewed in Perth. At times there seemed to be a different concept of space and privacy. Yet I could not help but think these communities, although maybe not ideal in terms of housing conditions, held a mirror up to the many things which we in the west may have lost in our communities, as we rush about in the hustle and bustle of our busy lives.

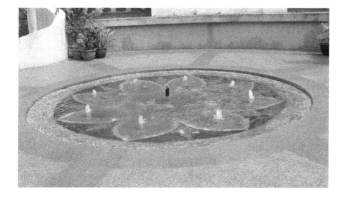

Photograph 8 The water feature at the Bali memorial in Kuta

The Kingsley Football Club reflections

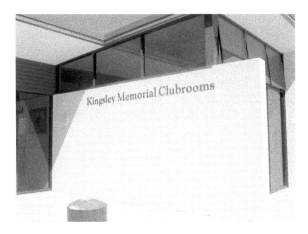

Photograph 9 The Kingsley Football Club memorial rooms [built in memory of Dean Gallagher, Byron Hancock, Corey Paltridge, David Ross, Anthony Stewart, Jason Stokes and Jonathan Wade]

'Forever in our thoughts – forever in our hearts'

The players from Kingsley Football Club who returned from Bali bruised and injured both physically and psychologically committed themselves to building memorial clubrooms in memory of their seven mates, and donations poured in from members of the public, the Kingsley community, builders and Perth entrepreneurs. Eventually the Kingsley memorial clubrooms were built, with much effort from many of the groups listed. The rooms were an attachment to an existing building and opened in 2003. This is the part of the clubrooms (photograph above) built in memory of the seven young footballers who lost their lives in the Bali bombing of 2002, and the phrase above is inscribed on the wall. It is a place where, on 12 October every year since the bombing, family, friends and the community gather to honour the young men who lost their lives, and a place where the survivors can meet with a shared understanding of what happened in Bali. It is an event I wait to be invited to each year, as in reality my support role is greatly reduced each year, and I now feel I am just part of the club family. It is an honour to be part of this gathering each year.

The room pictured above is a lovely quiet area of tribute away from the hustle and bustle of the busy clubrooms. The most poignant part of the tribute is the photographs of the seven smiling and happy-looking young men on the wall. On each anniversary the memorial area (pictured) and the main clubroom are mostly filled with the same familiar faces, all of whom share a common bond, including members of the committee, friends and family members of those killed and injured, the general public, and of course the young men who survived the bombing and some other players from the footy club.

A number of the young men now bring their wives and children, and it has become quite a family affair. Sometimes a footy (football) is produced and an informal kickabout happens, or people gather in groups for a chat, a cup of tea or a beer and some snacks provided by the committee. As an indication of how important the event is, I spoke a few years back to a couple from the Eastern States who were in Perth on holiday. They had a family member who been injured in the bombing and felt they just wanted to be there to be part of the anniversary tribute and be with people who would understand. They knew no one at the club, yet I have a feeling they made many friends that day, as they were generously welcomed.

There are perhaps fewer tears shed now (at times these included mine, usually after the event) and maybe fewer members of the general public attending. Overall less support or advice is needed from myself and others. People have moved on with their lives, married, had children, moved away from the area, moved overseas, etc., yet this does not mean people have forgotten the seven young men or the enormity and tragedy of what happened. The area to the left of the photograph is where most people walk along at some point in the day to look at the young men's photographs and cases of memorabilia from the Sari club site (right of photograph), or sit quietly looking out at the memorial rose garden and statue. They sit in quiet tribute, alone with their thoughts, or someone will, with unspoken permission, often join them in quiet reflection; there are hugs and tears are often shed. The committee members who open up the clubrooms each year on 12 October have vowed to continue to open them for as long as people want to meet on the anniversary. It is a privilege to attend.

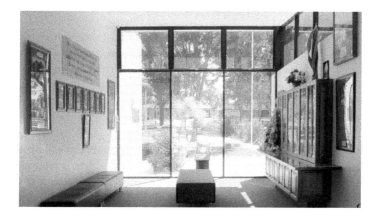

Photograph 10 The memorial rooms

The candlelight vigil

A total of 202 people died in the Bali bombing of 2002. Of these, 88 were Australians, seven of whom were members of the footy club in Kingsley. Dean Gallagher, Byron Hancock, Corey Paltridge, David Ross, Anthony Stewart, Jason Stokes and Jonathan Wade lost their lives that evening. Their names, family members, friends and the football community would become familiar to me both then and over the years in which I have been involved.

I initially heard the news as I was working from home on the Monday following the bombing. It was reported on the morning news, and I quickly stopped the mundane housework I was attending to and sat watching in horror what had happened. I decided I would volunteer my services as a psychologist, with skills that would perhaps be useful. After a roundabout search for the telephone number of anyone involved, I called one of the club committee members. He was deeply shocked by what had happened and he invited me to attend a community and club meeting later that evening. Little did I know how deeply I would get involved and how deeply my involvement would affect my life.

Over the course of the first few months and up to a year later, there would be many meetings that I and many others would attend in this volunteer role. I joined the co-ordinating committee, with meetings to organise getting the young men home, late-night phone calls to help get injured men home from the Eastern States, meetings to try and decide how to handle and properly handle the many monetary donations that were flooding in, meetings to consider what support could we offer and what was appropriate; these are just a few that I recall.

Between meetings I offered individual and group support work in person and on the telephone. By instinct (and, when I had time, research) rather than training I tried to gain people's respect, gave very basic support and a 'listening ear', validated the victims' feelings, which seemed to help, and made and took many, many phone calls. It was difficult at times to hear a number of first and sometimes second-hand victims' stories following such a traumatic event. The retelling of stories was not something I invited; however, many times – understandably – the victims wanted to tell them, almost in an effort to 'get it out' – sometimes because they felt they had to protect others and my rooms and other venues were, thankfully, a place where they could safely let go if they wanted to. Although this was a small part of my volunteer role, it was a period of time which they and I would recall for the rest of our lives. Yet I could not and would not ever compare my emotions, my fatigue, my loss of time and of family time to the enormity of their experiences and loss. Mine paled into insignificance.

In between I tried to manage my counselling business and family life without feeling too guilty (that was difficult). My family and friends were so supportive; I can't thank them enough. I was not alone – many other people, too numerous to mention, came together to help the football club at that time, and we helped each other and did the best we could. We sometimes learned on the job, as after all no one had ever been involved in this type of work before. We made mistakes, we hopefully learned from them, and everyone eventually understood. Many quiet tears were shed and the committee meetings sometimes became a mixture of emotions and, yes, sometimes understandable anger. Bonds were formed and a quiet understanding evolved regarding what had to be done, whatever it took.

There were many memorable moments that I can recall. One in particular comes to mind as everyone's efforts culminated in a candlelit vigil conducted by the late Father Brian Morrison. Around 300 people were expected to attend; in the end 3,000 people turned up to show their support. Looking out at the sea of faces on that night it was lovely to see a show of solidarity and the community spirit so often not seen. The vigil gave comfort to grieving families, the injured, their friends and the community. One young man had been confirmed dead and quite a number were still missing. Donations were given to the fund for the families and the clubrooms. I recall a male member of the public – a university lecturer, who was clearly upset – coming up to me with a donation, placing it in my hand and donating in honour of one of his ex-uni students, who had been killed in the bombing. He talked a little of his memory of the young man (I am sadly unable to recall his name) and what a fine young man he was.

An eternal flame was lit on the night and would stay lit until all of the fine young men, the missing players, were returned home. The candle is now on view in one of the memorabilia glass cases pictured. The lives of everyone involved in the response would change for ever. Invaluable lessons about life and the brutality of strangers in a distant war would occur, along with the most important lessons and knowledge about the beauty and kindness of strangers in two different countries who helped the young men and their families in so many ways.

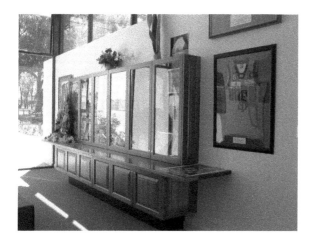

Photograph 11 Memorabilia glass cases at the Kingsley memorial

The bravery of the young men who searched the morgues and hospitals for their young friends, lost forever. Their first-hand accounts are held deep in my memory for ever and I am in awe of them. I am proud to know them, their families and the Kingsley Football Club community. It was and still is a huge privilege to be involved, and I am grateful for the support they gave the initial project.

Index

For Product Safety Concerns and Information please contact our EU
representative GPSR@taylorandfrancis.com
Taylor & Francis Verlag GmbH, Kaufingerstraße 24, 80331 München, Germany

www.ingramcontent.com/pod-product-compliance
Ingram Content Group UK Ltd.
Pitfield, Milton Keynes, MK11 3LW, UK
UKHW020954180425
457613UK00019B/670